The Self in Performance

Susana Pendzik • Renée Emunah • David Read Johnson
Editors

The Self in Performance

Autobiographical, Self-Revelatory, and Autoethnographic Forms of Therapeutic Theatre

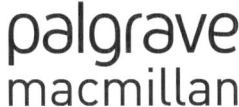

Editors
Susana Pendzik
Drama Therapy Graduate Program
Tel Hai Academic College
Upper Galilee, Israel

Renée Emunah
California Institute of Integral Studies
San Francisco, USA

David Read Johnson
Institute for Developmental
Transformations
New Haven, Connecticut, USA

ISBN 978-1-349-71259-5   ISBN 978-1-137-53593-1   (eBook)
DOI 10.1057/978-1-137-53593-1

Library of Congress Control Number: 2016955185

Cover image © Roger Bamber / Alamy Stock Photo
Cover design by Will Speed

Printed on acid-free paper

This Palgrave Macmillan imprint is published by Springer Nature
The registered company is Nature America Inc.
The registered company address is: 1 New York Plaza, New York, NY 10004, U.S.A.

PREFACE

This book was born out of misunderstanding. When Susana proposed to
Renée and David that we compile a book on therapeutic autobiographical,
self-revelatory, ethnographic performance, there was immediate agreement. When we met to discuss our prospective project, we quickly realized we did not share the same definitions of these labels. Worse, after
more debate, we lost confidence in our own views of these labels. Review
of the literature convinced us even further that there was a lack of clarity
about the concepts, boundaries, and practices of the self in performance.
Paradoxically, this proved to us the necessity for the book: to gather a
collection of work, and then to make initial efforts to map out the topog-
raphy of this field. In so doing, we discovered that an entirely unique
branch of drama therapy performance has been developing over the past
thirty years, and that now is the time for it to be properly identified. The
three of us had strenuous conversations that challenged each of our previously held assumptions. We have each grown from these encounters. We
hope that you, the reader, do as well, for something powerful and healing
occurs when a person creates a performance based on their life. Why that
happens, and how that happens, is the subject of this book.

We would like to acknowledge the contributions of our authors and the
courage and creativity of the clients and students who have revealed their
lives in these performances. Susana would like to acknowledge the creators quoted in her chapter, as well as those who over the years, through
their experiences and performances, helped to elucidate a dramaturgical
approach. She is profoundly indebted to Dr. Chen Alon for his long-
standing partnership in accompanying Therapeutic Autobiographical

Performances and for his precious insights for this chapter, and to Galila Oren for her invaluable input and encouragement. Susana would also like to thank Tel Hai Academic College, and the Swiss Dramatherapy Institute for their support. Renée would like to acknowledge the many students and graduates of the Drama Therapy Program at the California Institute of Integral Studies who embraced the Self-Rev process, and over the years helped to deepen and expand the form. She is also grateful for the ongoing collaboration with her colleagues and fellow faculty in the Drama Therapy Program, especially Gary Raucher. David would like to acknowledge the members of the Developmental Transformations community who have been the inspiration and audience for his self-revelatory performances.

Drama Therapy Graduate Program,
Tel Hai Academic College, Israel   Susana Pendzik

California Institute of Integral Studies,
Drama Therapy Graduate Program
San Francisco, USA   Renée Emunah

Yale University, New Haven, Connecticut, USA   David Read Johnson

CONTENTS

NOTES ON CONTRIBUTORS

Prentiss Benjamin is a graduate of the Drama Therapy program at New York University, USA. She is also an actress, having performed Off-Broadway and in regional theatres across the country.

Drew Bird is a senior lecturer in the Dramatherapy Master's program, College of Health and Social Care, University of Derby, UK. Drew has worked as a dramatherapist in child and adolescent mental health, specializing in childhood trauma, adult mental health and palliative care, as well as in private practice. He is a solo performer, director and playback trainer.

Zeina Daccache is Founder and Director of Catharsis—Lebanese Center for Drama Therapy. Zeina has been implementing drama therapy processes in Lebanon and the Middle East since 2006. She has directed plays and films for advocacy and awareness-raising, including *12 Angry Lebanese—The Play* (2009) with male inmates in the Roumieh prison; *12 Angry Lebanese—The Documentary* (2009); *Scheherazade in Baabda—The Play* (2012) and *Scheherazade's Diary—The Documentary* (2013) with women inmates in the Baabda Prison. Zeina and the documentaries she directed have received awards for distinguished contributions to the field.

Ditty Dokter is Course Leader of the Dramatherapy Master's program, Anglia Ruskin University, UK, and Researcher at the Arts Therapies Research Centre KENVAK, Netherlands. Ditty previously held course leadership positions at the universities of Hertfordshire and Roehampton; her most recent clinical appointment was as Head of an Arts Therapies Department at an adult and older people's mental health trust. Her research interest is in intercultural practice. Her books include: *Arts Therapies and Clients with Eating Disorders* (1994); *Arts Therapists, Refugees and Migrants* (1998); *Supervision in Dramatherapy* (2008); *Dramatherapy and Destructiveness* (2011); and *Intercultural Arts Therapies Research* (in press).

Pam Dunne is Director of the Drama Therapy Institute of Los Angeles, USA, and Professor Emeritus of Music, Theatre & Dance Department at California State University, Los Angeles. The pioneer of Narradrama, Dr. Dunne's work includes the books, *Narrative Therapist and the Arts*; *Narradrama*; and *Double Stick Tape: Poetry, Photography, Drama and Narrative with Adolescents*, and the film, *Exploring Narradrama*. Dr. Dunne has conducted extensive international workshops, served as NADTA president, and is a founding member of its Board of Examiners. In 2014, Dr. Dunne was selected as the recipient of the NADTA Teaching Excellence Award.

Renée Emunah is Founder/Director of the graduate Drama Therapy Program at the California Institute of Integral Studies, USA, where she has been a professor for over 30 years. She is the author of the book *Acting for Real: Drama Therapy Process, Technique, and Performance* (1994) which has become a classic in the field, and has been translated into Chinese and Japanese. She is co-editor with David Johnson of *Current Approaches in Drama Therapy* (2009). She was on the Editorial Board of the international journal *Arts in Psychotherapy* over many years. She is the recipient of the North American Drama Therapy Association (NADTA) Gertrud Schattner Distinguished Award for Outstanding Contribution to the Field of Drama Therapy (1996). She is an international trainer; a pioneering practitioner in the field; the originator of Self-Revelatory Performance; and a past-President of the NADTA.

Alida Gersie is a Writer, Psychotherapist and Planned Change Consultant. She advises senior professionals in the arts, health and education on creative ways to improve the outcomes of their work. For many years Alida directed the Postgraduate Arts Therapies Programme at the University of Hertfordshire, UK. There she developed Britain's first MA in Dramatherapy, supervisor training courses, Europe-wide 'train the trainer' courses for adults with disabilities, and story-for-change modules. Since 2001 she has initiated arts-based public health initiatives. She is the author of several key books used by change agents in over 40 countries.

Dovrat Harel teaches at the Graduate School of Creative Arts Therapies, Haifa University, Israel. Dovrat, a drama therapist and supervisor in private practice, has been working for 17 years in day care centers with older adults, specializing in people with dementia and their families. She works with the Alzheimer's Association of Israel (EMDA), developing programs of creative care for people with cognitive decline. In 2011 Dovrat was honored with an award for her doctoral research on people with dementia by the International Institute for Reminiscence and Life Review (IIRLR), University of Wisconsin-Superior, USA.

Maria Hodermarska is Master Teacher of Drama Therapy, New York University, USA. Maria is a drama therapist and full-time faculty member in NYU's program in drama therapy. She has authored and co-authored many book chapters and essays on drama therapy. Currently, she works with young people from around the world who have lost a family member to an act of extremism or armed conflict and is developing a theater project with her son and several colleagues examining how disability performs.

Jean-Francois Jacques is a dramatherapist and clinical supervisor both in private practice and a community adult mental health service, a community theatre director, and a researcher. He is an invited lecturer of the MA program in Dramatherapy at Anglia Ruskin University, UK, where he teaches autobiographical research and is studying the co-creation of meaning in autobiographical performance in dramatherapy.

David Read Johnson is Director, Institute for Developmental Transformations; Co-Director, Post Traumatic Stress Center, New Haven, CT, USA; Associate Clinical Professor, Department of Psychiatry, Yale University School of Medicine; co-editor (with Renee Emunah), *Current Approaches in Drama Therapy* (2009); co-editor (with Susana Pendzik and Stephen Snow), *Assessment in Drama Therapy* (2012); co-editor (with Nisha Sajnani), *Trauma-Informed Drama Therapy* (2014); Past President, North American Drama Therapy Association; and Past Editor-in-Chief, *Arts in Psychotherapy*.

Stephanie Omens is a licensed Creative Arts Therapist in New York State, USA, Registered Drama Therapist and certified Child Life Specialist. Stephanie has worked at Hackensack University Medical Center since 2002 with chronically ill hospitalized, bereaved and prematurely born infants and children, and is an adjunct instructor at the Department of

Drama, Tisch School of the Arts, New York University, where she teaches drama therapy. Stephanie is co-author of a chapter in *The Health Professions: Trends and Opportunities in U.S. Health Care* (2007), and is author of a chapter in *Trauma Informed Drama Therapy: Transforming Clinics, Classrooms and Communities* (2014).

Susana Pendzik is Head of the Graduate Program in Drama Therapy at Tel Hai Academic College, Israel, also lecturing at the Theatre Studies Department of the Hebrew University of Jerusalem, and at the Dramatherapy Institute in Switzerland. She conducts workshops world-wide, and is pioneering drama therapy in Latin America. She has taught autobiographical therapeutic performance for over 20 years, and is the author of numerous papers and chapters, a handbook of group work with abused women (1992 in Spanish and 1995 in German), and co-editor of *Assessment in Drama Therapy* (2012) with David Johnson and Stephen Snow.

Jules Dorey Richmond and **David Richmond** are both Senior Lecturers in Theatre & Performance at York St John University, UK, where for the past ten years Jules has been teaching autobiographical solo performance, and David has been running a module 'Artist as Witness' which begins with a pilgrimage to Auschwitz and ends with a collaborative ensemble performance. They have been collaborating partners for over 25 years, creating works in diverse contexts, pulling together their respective disciplines of visual art and theatre. Their research on memory, place and performance can be traced in both their solo projects and collaborative practice, most notably in their Theatre of Witness series of works with veterans, witnesses and survivors of WW2, documented in *Performance Research: On Trauma*.

Sheila Rubin is a drama therapist, storyteller and marriage and family therapist in private practice in San Francisco and Berkeley. She has directed over 25 self-revelatory performances of CIIS students as their final project, and five of her own, as well as hundreds of shorter Embodied Life-Stories performances. She teaches self-revelatory performance directing and healing shame workshops for therapists internationally. She has written several chapters, among them, 'Self-revelatory performance' in *Interactive and Improvisational Drama* (2007); and 'Almost magic' in *The Use of Expressive Arts Therapy in Treating Depression* (2015).

Nisha Sajnani is Associate Professor and Coordinator of the Graduate Drama Therapy Program at Lesley University, USA. Nisha also holds faculty appointments in the Harvard Program in Refugee Trauma, and New York University's Drama Therapy Program, is the Editor of the *Drama Therapy Review*, and a past-president of the North American Drama Therapy Association. She has authored numerous publications on improvisation, diversity, arts-based research, trauma, and critical theory. She is also the artistic director of *Theatre Beyond Borders* and co-coordinator of the Expressive Therapies Research Center at Lesley University.

Anna Seymour is Senior Lecturer in Dramatherapy, University of Roehampton, UK. Anna is a dramatherapist, academic, and researcher. She is a Principal Fellow of the Higher Education Academy and has presented conference papers, master classes and delivered training across Britain and internationally. She is Editor of the peer-reviewed British Association of Dramatherapists journal, *Dramatherapy*, and Series Editor of *Dramatherapy: Approaches, Relationships, Critical Ideas*.

Stephen Snow is Professor of Drama Therapy in the Department of Creative Arts Therapies and Co-Director of Research at The Centre for the Arts in Human Development, Concordia University, Montreal, Quebec, Canada. Stephen is an actor, director and drama therapist with thirty years of experience in many clinical and educational settings. As an actor, he has performed in over 100 theatre productions, including experimental theatre in the 1970s and two self-revelatory pieces, *Seething Brains* and *Nightride in the City*. He has written many articles and chapters on drama therapy and is the co-editor of two books, *Assessment in the Creative Arts Therapies* (2009) and *Assessment in Drama Therapy* (2012).

Armand Volkas is an associate professor at California Institute of Integral Studies, USA, Drama Therapy Program. Armand is a psychotherapist, drama therapist and theatre director. He is Clinical Director of the Living Arts Counseling Center, and Director of the Living Arts Playback Theatre Ensemble, now in its 28th year. Armand has developed innovative international programs using drama therapy for social change, intercultural conflict transformation and peace-building, and has worked with autobiographic therapeutic theatre for many years.

Gideon Zehavi is a lecturer and PhD candidate in the Theatre Studies Department at the Hebrew University of Jerusalem, Israel, and adjunct faculty at the Drama Therapy Program of Tel Hai Academic College,

Israel. Gideon is a drama therapist and supervisor, who works internationally, co-leads the Institute for Developmental Transformations in Israel, is currently researching therapeutic autobiographical performances, and has written several papers on drama therapy with the autistic spectrum disorder population.

CHAPTER 1

The Self in Performance: Context, Definitions, Directions

Susana Pendzik, Renée Emunah,
and David Read Johnson

During the second half of the twentieth century, performance and artistic expression took a strong turn toward the personal with the embrace of the memoir in literature, sociopolitical and feminist visual art, solo

S. Pendzik, PhD, MA, RDT (✉)
Tel Hai Academic College, Kiryat Shemona, Israel

Hebrew University of Jerusalem, Jerusalem, Israel

Swiss Institute of Dramatherapy, St Gallen, Switzerland
e-mail: pend@netvision.net.il

R. Emunah, PhD, RDT-BCT
California Institute of Integral Studies, San Francisco, CA, USA
e-mail: remunah@ciis.edu

D.R. Johnson, PhD, RDT-BCT
Institute for Developmental Transformations, New York, NY, USA
Post Traumatic Stress Center, New Haven, CT, USA
Department of Psychiatry, Yale University School of Medicine, New Haven, CT, USA
e-mail: davidreadjohnson@gmail.com

© The Author(s) 2016
S. Pendzik et al. (eds.), *The Self in Performance,*
DOI 10.1057/978-1-137-53593-1_1

1

performance art, and autobiographical performance. Since the start of the twenty-first century, with the pervasive public interest in reality television, YouTube and iPhone selfies, the private has indeed become public. As a result, the boundaries between truth and fiction, the real and the dramatic, have never been so ambiguous; the self can be viewed as being performed, everywhere.

Within the field of theatre, this impulse has expressed itself in the emergence of what might be called *self-referential* or *personal* theatre—that is, theatre in which the content of the performance consists of material from the actual lives of the performers. This work can be loosely categorized into *autobiographical* forms (concerning the actor's personal life) and *autoethnographic* forms (concerning the actor's ethnicity, class, gender, or social grouping). Within each of these can be differentiated *nontherapeutic* forms (where the aim is primarily artistic, educational, or advocacy), and *therapeutic* forms (where the aim is personal growth). This book is about this last category: autobiographical and autoethnographical therapeutic theatre/performance.

The idea that therapeutic practice correlates with the telling of personal stories has a deep hold on western thinking. But when does telling one's story have a liberating effect, and when does it become merely a recounting of one's misery and victimization? This question acquires further significance in the context of autobiographical performance, as rehearsal practices allow experiences to become more rooted in our bodies and brains, and exposure in front of an audience helps to validate them. Does performing life experiences, obsessions, memories or dreams on stage invariably bring about therapeutic results? (Pendzik, 2013a; Thompson, 2009). What is required for an autobiographical performance to fulfill the function of promoting psychological well-being, healing from trauma, or advancing personal growth?

Psychoanalyst Charles Rycroft (1983) has questioned the therapeutic potential of autobiographical writings that merely serve the purpose of 'advertising the continued existence of a long-standing ego' (p. 193). He emphasizes the need for therapeutic autobiography to involve a reflexive practice that aims at self-discovery. In a true therapeutic process, he says, 'a dialectic takes place between present "I" and past "me," at the end of which both have changed and the author-subject could say equally truthfully, "I wrote it" and "It wrote me."' (p. 192).

The potentially empowering or healing effects often attributed to autobiographical performances may be associated with the feminist and political inception of the genre, which fueled the sense of personal agency exercised by the authors/performers, underlined the transformative possibilities inherent in the act of storying our lives, and offered a place of centrality—literally, a stage—to uncanonical, radical, and public representations of the personal (Claycomb, 2012; Heddon, 2008; Park-Fuller, 2003; Spry, 2011).

In this introductory chapter we begin by contextualizing therapeutic self-referential performance in the framework of other self-referential modes (western and non-western), connecting and contrasting it with parallel developments, particularly in autobiographical and autoethnographic theatre, that do not emphasize a therapeutic aim. The chapter lays out various definitions proposed by scholars and practitioners, highlighting common concepts as well as discussing areas that lack clarity. Throughout, we attempt to articulate the complex relationships between theatrical and therapeutic aims in such performances. After briefly summarizing the essence of each chapter in this book, we conclude by offering suggestions for future research.

SELF-REFERENTIAL ARTISTIC MODALITIES IN NON-WESTERN AND WESTERN TRADITIONS

Historically, the use of self-referential modes as a tool for personal expression that is both introspective and artistically crafted goes back centuries, and has been practiced throughout the world. As Jane Walker (1994) asserts, 'All civilizations, not just the western, are attentive and have been attentive throughout their history to…"individual self-understanding"' (p. 207)—including Chinese, Japanese, Indian, Arabic, and other non-western traditions, in which aesthetic self-referential forms have been cultivated by both women and men. For example, the Japanese literary tradition since its onset contains self-reflective works that can be viewed as having an autobiographical intent (Walker, 1994); among these, the *Japanese poetic diary* that flourished throughout the eleventh century, was considered to be 'in its highest aesthetic quality, the property of women' (Miner, 1968, p. 42). Closer to a performance of the self are the autobiographical narratives of the Kayabi people (an indigenous group living in the Brazilian state of Mato Grosso), who interweave accounts of their personal experiences in the context of their rituals—including shamanic cures, in which shamans present their own dreams, emotional states, and former cosmic travels as part of their performative healing methods (Oakdale, 2005).

Autobiographical narratives in non-western traditions may exhibit more stylized or fictionalized versions of the self (Walker, 1994), multiple and hybrid images (such as the merging of self and context in Frida Kahlo's self-portraits (Helland, 1992), or may defy organization 'around a privileged Self, in relation to which events and other persons are arranged as background' (More-Gilbert, 2009, p. 103). As noted by postcolonial and feminist critics, marginalized artists may voice their self-narratives in forms that privilege plurality, emphasize orality, or use dialogical forms, rather than the traditional western self-presentation or confessional style (Miller, Taylor, & Carver, 2003; Smith & Watson, 1998).

Grace (2003) highlights that in western culture, textual narratives tend to dominate the critical discourse as an organizing axis for understanding all forms of autobiographical representations. Scholarship traditionally grants Saint Augustine's *Confessions* a position of fatherhood, placing it as 'the origin of modern western autobiography' (Anderson, 2011, p. 17). Aligned with his work are a host of male descendants (such as Rousseau and Wordsworth) who have been considered exemplary in the genre, despite the fact that life-writing has been used by many female authors (such as Saint Teresa of Avila) as a strategy to gain access to the written word through one of the few channels that were open to women: writing about their personal experiences (Weber, 1990). The western literary canon has taken a mostly ambivalent stance regarding self-referential writing, either questioning its literary merit or restricting its focus to illustrious (usually male) representatives. Critical debate has centered for the most part on establishing the author's honesty and truthfulness in autobiographical works, memoirs, and other forms of self-writing, and in discussing the relationship between author and text (Anderson, 2011; De Man, 1979; Smith & Watson, 1998).

CONTEXTUALIZING SELF-REFERENTIAL THEATRE AND ITS RELATION TO THERAPEUSIS

In contrast to the long-established patriarchal approach to self-referential written texts, it appears that *self-referential performed praxes* in all their shapes and forms have been born in freedom: A gender and politically-aware perspective has been adopted in the critical discourse of self-referential theatre, supporting self-determination, promoting emancipatory actions, challenging colonization, shaping a critical awareness, and endorsing a feminist worldview that reveals the in/visible threads linking the personal and the public (Forte, 1988; Schmor, 1994). As Deidre Heddon (2008) claims:

> The autobiographical and the political are interconnected. Who speaks? What is spoken? What sorts of lives are represented, contested, imagined? The vast majority of autobiographical performances have been concerned with using the public arena of performance in order to 'speak out,' attempting to make visible denied or marginalized subjects, or to 'talk back,' aiming to challenge, contest, and problematize dominant representations about those subjects (p. 20).

She adds that during the 1970s the main motivation for translating personal content 'into live performance was inarguably tied to consciousness-raising activities' (p. 21), which were meant to activate the collective understanding that personal life and gender oppression should be explored together. In the last decades of the twentieth century, this spirit reverberated in the celebratory performances of queer autobiographical solos, which challenged social invisibility and marginalization, exploring issues of identity and 'speaking out' (Sandhal, 2003; Pearlman, 2015).

Heddon (2008) defines the current work of autobiographical performance as one that aims 'to explore (question, reveal) the relationship between the personal and the political, engaging with and theorizing the discursive construction of selves and experience' (p. 162). In her view, by bringing 'to the fore the self as a performed role,' autobiographical performance reveals 'not only the multiplicity of the performing subject, but also the multiplicity of discourses that work to forge subjects' (p. 39).

In a similar vein, autoethnographic theatre methods are context-oriented and informed by socio/political/gender approaches (Saldaña, 2003; Spry, 2001); they tend to 'have a social awareness agenda' (Saldaña, 2011 p. 31) and to address issues such as gender and racial inequity (Spry, 2010). Conceived as politically and academically transgressive forms of inquiry, these methods aim at re/introducing the body into research discourse in a way that 'can emancipate the scholarly voice from the monostylistic confines of academic discourse' (Spry 2001, p. 720). In Tami Spry's (2011) words:

Performative autoethnography is a *personal/political social praxis*, and a critically reflexive methodology, meaning it provides a framework to critically reflect upon the ways in which our personal lives intersect, collide, and commune with others in the body politic in ways alternate to hegemonic cultural expectations. It provides a narrative apparatus to pose and engage the questions of our global lives, asking us to embrace one another as fully as we challenge one another. (p. 54)

It is in this context that self-referential theatre methods come to intersect with therapeutic practices, as personal inquiry and critical self-reflection are pursued in connection with topics such as identity, agency, empowerment, emancipatory/oppressive self-representations, memory, and narrative (Langellier & Peterson, 2004)—which have traditionally been the foci of psychotherapy and psychology. An implicit, almost natural alliance is thus forged between self-referential theatre forms and therapeutic processes.

Scholars from the fields of both theatre and drama therapy have acknowledged that self-referential performances can have therapeutic side benefits (Emunah, 2015). Heddon (2008) recognizes that autobiographical performances 'may equate with personal healing,' by referring to works by artists like Spalding Gray and Linda Montano that deal with traumatic life events as 'acts of recovery' (p. 54). She notes the therapeutic potential of pieces such as Linda Park-Fuller's *A clean breast of it*, which the performer defined as an act of personal and political agency that helped her to transform her subjective identity from the 'prescribed... role of "patient-victim"' into that of a survivor (Park-Fuller, 2003, p. 215). Yet many of these scholars and performers hesitate to identify their work as therapeutic, underscoring a common confusion about whether expressing emotion or revealing personal information necessarily lies within a therapeutic domain. Noting the emotional impact of self-reflective performed autoethnography, Spry (2011) cautions that 'emotion is not inherently epistemic' (p. 108):

Performance studies practitioners have worked with the embodiment of emotion in the production of knowledge for centuries, and are aware of the potential dangers when expecting the expression of emotion in research to stand-in for aesthetic acumen. (p. 108)

The intersection between self-referential performance as an art form and as a therapeutic method therefore is both a place of meeting and of departure. Emunah (2015) notes, 'Autobiographical theatre... involves dramatic storytelling or dramatization of personal life material, but without a conscious aim of transforming or healing this material' (p. 72); on the other hand, what she terms *self-revelatory performance* is both a therapeutic process and a form of theatre. She states:

> An aesthetically portrayed revealing and reweaving of a core and current issue in the performer's life can be compelling, if not riveting, to an audience. The natural suspense and unpredictability in the unfolding of the piece, along with the immediacy of real issues being grappled with in new ways, are all ingredients for good theatre. (Emunah, 2015, p. 79)

Richard Schechner (2013) uses the concept of the *efficacy–entertainment dyad* to differentiate between ritual and theatre (both being performances): When the primary purpose is effecting change, the efficacy aspect is highlighted, whereas when aesthetics are the primary goal, the entertainment factor prevails. Schechner (2013) encourages us to see the relationship between efficacy and entertainment not as a rigid dyad 'but as a braid or helix, tightening and loosening over time and in specific cultural contexts' (p. 80). We are in agreement: aesthetics and therapeusis are not mutually exclusive; more often than not, they powerfully coincide (Emunah, 1994, 2015; Emunah & Johnson, 1983; Pendzik, 2013a, 2013b; Sajnani, 2012; Snow, D'Amico, & Tanguay, 2003).

DEFINITIONS AND TERMINOLOGY

Self-referential forms tend to call themselves by a plethora of names. According to Smith and Watson (2010), the 'rich and diverse history of self-referential modes requires that we make some crucial distinctions among key terms—*autobiography, memoir, life writing, life narrative*—that may seem to imply the same thing' (p. 2). And there are more terms, including *testimonial, autoethnography* and *psychobiography*. A similar nomenclatorial overabundance applies to self-referential theatre and performance. Researching the genres of *ethnotheatre* and *ethnodrama*, Saldaña (2011) discovered over 80 unique terms for the form, including: *autodrama, autoperformance, everyday life performance, factual theatre, generative autobiography, heritage theatre, memory theatre, mystory, reality theatre, performing autobiography, reminiscence theatre, self-performance, and testimonial theatre* (pp. 13–14). More names could enrich this list— especially in referring to autobiographical performance: *autobiographical storytelling performance* (Langellier & Peterson, 2004), *confessional performance* (Schmor, 1994), *self-story* (Beglau, 2012), *solo autobiographical performance* (Wallace, 2006), and *theatre of the real* (Martin, 2013). Some names consider the place where the performance takes place as having biographical agency, thus adding terms such as autobiographical site-specific performance or *autopography* (Stephenson, 2012).

A similar multiplicity for describing performances of the self is present within the field of drama therapy—sometimes informed by culture, language, and practice-related factors. Renée Emunah (1994, 2015) conceived and developed self-revelatory performance (Self-Rev), a form of drama therapy and theatre that has been practiced predominantly in the USA and Canada. In her words, 'Self-Revelatory Performance is a form of drama therapy and theatre in which a performer creates an original theatrical piece out of the raw material of current life issues' (Emunah, 2015, p. 71). The focus is on multi-leveled strands of healing, which ultimately augment (rather than compromise) theatrical quality. Her descriptions of therapeutic performance, and particularly her analyses of methods of theatrically grappling with therapeutic issues, and of what constitutes healing in personal theatre, have influenced and informed the field as a whole regardless of terminology and form.

Many practitioners use the more generic term *autobiographical therapeutic theatre/performance* (ATP). Pendzik (2013a) defines autobiographical therapeutic theatre as a form of drama therapy that involves the development of a performance based on personal material, presented in front an audience, and is conceived with a therapeutic aim. She adds:

> Even such a broad definition already implies what it is not: It is not an improvised piece, but one that is developed over time, and is therefore subjected to a rehearsal phase; it is not centered on literary or universal works, but on personal experience; it has a communicative function: it is meant to be performed in front of other people, thus, taking their implicit presence into consideration. Finally, it is not made for entertainment ends, but there is a therapeutic aspect at play. The combination of these premises also indicates the existence of a balance between *process* and *product*—one which is indispensable to keep; for in autobiographical therapeutic theatre both ends of the rope are equally important. (pp. 4–5)

In the United Kingdom, performances about the self that dramatherapy students are required to create during their training have been called *personal theatre* (Seymour, Chap. 14), or simply autobiographical performances. Jacques (Chap. 7) speaks of *autobiographical performance in dramatherapy*, while Dokter and Gersie (Chap. 13) note that these as well as other terms have been used interchangeably in the UK.

Despite the subtle distinctions between the names many of our chapter contributors apply to their work, we recommend the term *autobiographical (or autoethnographic) therapeutic performance* (or *theatre*) (ATP) as the generic, overarching label for this work, and will therefore use it throughout this book. Although Emunah brought her concept of Self-Rev into being before many began to use the term autobiographical therapeutic performance, in the end, Self-Rev is a more specific form with its own criteria - given its emphasis on exploring current personal issues, on a depth of therapeutic *working through*, and on a high degree of artistic mastery. Although overlapping with or informed by Self-Rev, some of the forms under ATP's broader umbrella emphasize specific aspects pertaining to the author's method of drama therapy or focus within clinical practice—as in Dunne's *Restoried Script Performance* (Chap. 10), or Volkas (Chap. 8), who finds the word *therapeutic* to be indispensable in describing the purpose of his work to potential clients.

OVERVIEW OF BOOK

The book is conceptually grounded in the intersection between theatre/performance and psychotherapy, moving fluidly between these paradigms; in some chapters concepts from other related disciplines are also incorporated.

Part I provides historical background and conceptual perspectives underlying current practice in ATP. Stephen Snow examines how experimental and avant-garde theatre influenced the development of Self-Rev—beginning with 'the demolition of the famous fourth wall of illusionistic theatre.' He elucidates how Artaud, Grotowski, The Living Theatre, The Open Theatre, and the autoperformance of Spaulding Gray were significant precedents to Self-Rev. Renée Emunah takes the reader on a close-up tour of what occurs 'behind the scenes' in the process of developing a Self-Rev (including the intensive collaboration between performer and director), followed by an analysis of what takes place for the performer in facing an audience—along with the role played by the audience—in such intimate theatrical productions. She emphasizes the centrality of *working through*, a process of engaging, developing, and transforming personal conflicts through embodied, theatrical means during rehearsal and performance phases. She then addresses the potential 'elephant' in the theatre with this kind of performance: the risk of self-indulgence.

Susana Pendzik outlines the dramaturgical elements involved in autobiographical therapeutic performance, focusing on what makes the presentation of personal stories move from a mere recounting of victimization to a therapeutic experience. Drawing on ideas in the work of Eugenio Barba, and exploring recurrent patterns that characterize the process as well as the performance pieces, she points out some archetypal configurations in ATPs, and offers examples of dramaturgical structures that turn the process into a therapeutic one. David Read Johnson then examines the experience of *surprise* in Self-Rev and considers the question: How does the performer achieve discovery on stage, when the piece has already been rehearsed and memorized? Johnson stresses the significance of Otherness in these personal creations, arising from the actor's unconscious, the director, stagecraft, and the presence of the audience. Relying on the instability theory in *Developmental Transformations*, he underscores the importance of the actor's vulnerability and openness to the present moment during the performance.

Nisha Sajnani also highlights the significance of others in solo performance, and explores the performance of personal story through the perspective of *relational aesthetics*. Her chapter elucidates a relational view of art, ethics, and audience. Incorporating examples of the works of several performance artists, Sajnani emphasizes the relationships that are inherent in both the process and content of personal theatre pieces, as well as between performer and audience. From the theoretical perspective of *intersubjectivity*, Jean-Francois Jacques continues the exploration of the relationship between performer and audience—a distinct theme throughout this book. Integrating elements from performance studies, drama therapy, phenomenology and intersubjectivity theory, he examines the dynamic encounter between actor and spectator. Jacques suggests a conceptual framework for the production of meaning, outlining layers and types of witnessing inherent in autobiographical performance in drama therapy.

Part II begins with presentations of ATP based on a range of approaches. Armand Volkas blends Joseph Campbell's concept of the *hero's journey*, anthropological models of *rites of passage*, and Eric Berne's *Transactional*

Analysis, into a process for helping clients create ATPs within a psycho-therapy practice. Sheila Rubin focuses on Self-Rev in healing shame and trauma. Her *Embodied Life Stories* process stresses the therapeutic relationship in helping to repair damaged or disrupted interpersonal bonds. Like Volkas, she highlights the importance of the reparative witness in accessing deeper aspects or new dimensions of the story. Pam Dunne's *Restoried Script Performance* process is based on Narrative Therapy and Positive Psychology, and, like Volkas and Rubin, is typically utilized with psychotherapy clients. The focus is on revealing problematic patterns or scripts in the client's life, and *re-storying* these to produce a more positive outcome or identity, presenting these transformations in the performance.

Drew Bird applies Clark Moustakas' six phases of *heuristic research* to the process of creating ATP, incorporating reflections from his own personal performance piece. The phases of engagement, immersion, incubation, illumination, explication, and creative synthesis provide a developmental framework for understanding the process of preparing ATPs. Examining four contemporary and recognized autobiographical performances in Israel, two of which were developed drama-therapeutically, Gideon Zehavi uses John Austin's concept of the *performative* within performance theory to examine the dynamics of transformative moments of presence that occur within autobiographical performances. He concludes that often these moments occur when the actor breaks out of role and briefly confronts the audience as him/herself, not unlike Johnson's conclusion that working through occurs when the discrepancy between the actor and his role is revealed to the audience.

The next two chapters focus on the use of personal theatre performances as part of dramatherapy (British spelling) training programs, specifically in the United Kingdom. Ditty Dokter and Alida Gersie review the history of autobiographical performance in British dramatherapy programs, and convey their content analysis of a set of performances as recollected by their alumni. Key themes of family relationships, diversity, being witnessed, privacy, and transformation are discussed, overlapping with some of the issues identified by Pendzik and others. Anna Seymour also interviews graduates about their personal theatre performances, and analyzes them from a dialectical, sociopolitical perspective, relying on Brecht and on Jacques Rancière's study of the power relations between performer and witness/audience. Her analysis reveals the multilayered and contradictory impulses within the actor (e.g., wanting to be seen and to hide from view), and raises questions about the nature of the audience's role in autobiographical performance.

The book then turns to more specific applications in Dovrat Harel's and Zeina Daccache's chapters on directing ATPs with particular populations: Harel, in Israel, with elderly people who have dementia, and Daccache, with inmates in Lebanese prisons. Harel describes how ATP revives and preserves memories, consistent with research on reminiscence within narrative gerontology. She illustrates how elderly clients improve their self-esteem and expand their positive self-identities. Daccache's work also empowers her clients to tell their life stories and dramatize their experiences in prison before large public audiences, building hope where there has been none. Inspired by Boal's *Legislative Theatre,* she relates her journey in using these performances to instigate social and legal reform in Lebanon, leading to the passage of a new law for 'The Protection of Women and Family Members from Domestic Violence,' approved by the Lebanese Parliament in 2014—a powerful demonstration of the potential of ATP to create tangible social change.

The final two chapters comprise descriptive accounts of collaborative personal performances by the creators of these pieces, who use the form in unique ways. Jules and David Richmond recount their process as a long-time couple of creating an autoethnographic performance exploring loss, aging, and the passage of time. Their poetic personal stories interface with their political commitment (and disillusion) with regard to urgent societal and ecological needs. Maria Hodermarska, Prentiss Benjamin, and Stephanie Omens turn the usual structure of ATP on its head by identifying the *play as the client.* In most performances, the actor is simultaneously the source of material, the playwright, and the performer. Hodermarska's team of drama therapists separates these roles entirely: there is no human client, and only the director links the performer, playwright, and the person who is the source of the personal material. Their reflections on this deconstructed process illuminate important themes and raise interesting questions in ATP and Self- Rev.

In our call for chapters we tried to reach a diversity of practitioners and scholars throughout the world, who may be using ATP or related forms of interventions; yet the reply came mainly from European, North American and Middle Eastern sources. We are therefore aware of the cultural and geographical limitations of the book, which will be addressed in future editions.

DISCUSSION

All of our contributors, as well as others engaged in autobiographical or autoethnographic therapeutic theatre, share core values and methods. The differences are mostly subtle, due to varying theoretical frameworks, specific needs of particular populations, settings and contexts, or simply preferred language of the author. All performances described in this book utilize or play with personal *narrative*. All utilize the fundamental power of personal *performance* before an *audience*, involving the *embodiment* of self while being *witnessed*. All emphasize the power of *revelation* of the performer and the corresponding ethics of *acceptance* on the part of the audience. These themes are deeply linked to the core tenets of both theatre and psychotherapy: the integration of mind and body; the centrality of the reparative relationship; and the complexity of connection and individuation of the person with regard to their history and cultural surround. Indeed, this work is born from, and reaches toward, freedom.

A number of issues deserve attention in future scholarship on ATP and its related forms. These include: (1) the role of the audience; (2) the role of the director/therapist; (3) use in drama therapy training; (4) the degree of creative license and its ethical dimension; (5) the impact of impending performance; and (6) the fact that ATPs are usually performed only once.

ROLE OF AUDIENCE

All of the authors in this volume reference the importance of the audience. They also imply that in these types of intimate, personal performances, the role of the audience is subtly different than that of standard theatre, linked to the fact that many in the audience are friends, colleagues, or family of the performer. Several authors hint at the ethical nature of this special relationship, though details are lacking. For example, how often and how thoroughly do practitioners conduct audience preparation prior to the performance, or de-briefing sessions or talks afterwards? If so, what is the content and purpose of these? Are they directed toward added benefit to the actor, or to the audience members? When, or in what contexts, would engaging the audience be advised, and when not? How do the expectations of the audience play a role?

Role of Director/Therapist

There is variation in the degree to which the director serves primarily as a therapist or drama therapist, or focuses more specifically on the artistic task of bringing an ATP to fruition. In the former case, the director may serve as the person's primary therapist long before and after the ATP, while in the latter, performer and director may collaborate only for the duration of the rehearsal and performance process. There is also variation in the degree to which the director/therapist privileges the therapeutic process versus ensuring that the final performance is of the best possible artistic quality. It is clear that some ATP directors/therapists prefer the consulting or witnessing role, while the main playwriting and material-generating tasks are accomplished by the performer; others are more active, taking charge of the shaping of the final script and intervening in the co-creative process. In Self-Rev, for example, the director is actively involved in both deepening the therapeutic possibilities and also in ensuring a product of theatrical excellence. How the trace of the director/therapist lives within the final performance as viewed by the audience remains an interesting question to explore.

Drama Therapy Training

A significant proportion of ATP practitioners work with drama therapy students in training programs, where ATP is encouraged or even required as a culminating project of their education. Most often fellow students as well as teachers are in the audience. Students/actors are asked to put forward a presentation of a highly personal nature, often as a capstone, which has an evaluative component. Many ethical and methodological issues arise that bear on the process of competition, evaluation, and power relations in the field. Though Emunah, Raucher, & Ramirez-Hernandez (2014), as well as Dokter and Gersie (Chap. 13), have provided us with the first data about this process, which shows that students value the experience highly and feel supported by the faculty and fellow students, not enough has been written about ATP in this setting.

CREATIVE LICENSE AND ETHICS

Most memoirs are allowed a certain degree of *creative license* to alter the names, places, actions, events, and even nature of the truth in the service of illuminating the meaning of the life of the person, or protecting anonymity. What is the relationship between truth and authenticity? This seems to be a central ethical issue in ATP, as in any memoir. Truth can be cloaked or revealed in metaphor and symbol, guided by a range of culturally based standards. Yet no author in this volume describes procedures to ensure ethical boundaries of representation in the ATP process, assuming perhaps that client/actors are being truthful about their lives. Much work can be done to study this process and integrate it with similar work being done in the field of autobiographical literature and autobiographical performance.

IMPACT OF THE IMPENDING PERFORMANCE

Several authors note the effect of having a date set for the performance on the rehearsal process in ATP. Indeed, this is an essential element of all theatre: opening night! As the day approaches, all sorts of decisions come to the fore—in producing, directing, and performing the piece– many of which could hardly be called therapeutic. Lines are cut, blocking is revamped. On the other hand, perhaps the deadline may propel clients to courageously go further and take risks they had been hesitant to before. How do actors and directors balance the aesthetic and therapeutic aims of ATP in these final, pressured moments?

A SINGLE PERFORMANCE?

In many cases, ATPs are performed only once. Why? Is this connected to the rite of passage implicit in the form? The anxiety generated by the task of ATP and its resolution upon completion, applause, and relief should not be misinterpreted as a successful resolution of the psychological wound itself. If these performances are deeply meaningful to both performers and audiences, then for them to be performed only once may represent a limitation in the possibilities of the form. For those who have taken their performance 'on the road,' what has their experience been? Do they continue to be therapeutic or do they shift toward standard (autobiographical) theatre? Again, we encourage the field to examine these issues in greater depth.

Summary

We hope this book will stimulate an active dialogue within and beyond the field of drama therapy regarding the fascinating and challenging work of autobiographical and autoethnographic therapeutic theatre and performance. This work has become central in most drama therapists' training and is progressively being applied in wider settings. It is intimately related to the broader fields of performance studies, as well as to postmodern and postcolonial literature, critical and feminist theory, and sociopolitical movements. It extends the therapeutic possibilities of drama therapy as a profession, and suggests new lines of inquiry into the nature of embodied, relational ethics. ATP is a form of drama therapy that belongs to the twenty-first century, and may indeed contribute to making that century a time of creative introspection and interconnection.

References

Anderson, L. (2011). *Autobiography*. Abingdon and New York: Routledge.

Beglau, N. (2012). *Self-story drama therapy: Healing through autobiographical stories in action*. Unpublished MA thesis, Pacifica Graduate Institute.

Claycomb, R. (2012). *Lives in play: Autobiography and biography on the feminist stage*. Ann Arbor: University of Michigan Press.

De Man, Paul. (1979). Autobiography as de-facement. *MLN, 94*(5), 919–930. http://links.jstor.org/sici?sici=0026-7910%28197912%2994%3A5%3C919%3AAAAD%3E2.0.CO%3B2-K

Emunah, R. (1994). *Acting for real: Drama therapy process, technique, and performance*. New York: Taylor & Francis.

Emunah, R. (2015). Self-revelatory performance. A form of drama therapy and theatre. *Drama Therapy Review, 1*(1), 71–85. https://doi.org/10.1386/dtr.1.1.71_1

Emunah, R., & Johnson, D. R. (1983). The impact of theatrical performance on the self-images of psychiatric patients. *Arts in Psychotherapy, 10*, 233–239.

Emunah, R., Raucher, G., & Ramirez-Hernandez, A. (2014). Self-revelatory performance in mitigating the impact of trauma. In N. Sajnani & D. Johnson (Eds.), *Trauma-informed drama therapy: Transforming clinics, classrooms, and communities* (pp. 93–121). Springfield, IL: Charles C Thomas.

Forte, J. (1988). Women's performance art: Feminism and postmodernism. *Theatre Journal, 40*(2), 217–235.

Grace, S. (2003). *Performing the auto/biographical pact: Towards a theory of identity in performance*. Accessed August 11, 2015, from http://www.english.ubc.ca/faculty/grace/thtr_ab.htm

Heddon, D. (2008). *Autobiography and performance*. Hampshire and New York: Palgrave Macmillan.

Helland, J. (1992). Culture, politics, and identity in the paintings of Frida Kahlo. In N. Broude & M. Garrard (Eds.), *The expanding discourse: Feminism and art history* (pp. 397–408). New York: HarperCollins.

Langellier, K., & Peterson, E. (2004). *Performing narrative: Storytelling in daily life*. Philadelphia: Temple University Press.

Martin, C. (2013). *Theatre of the real*. Basingstoke and New York: Palgrave Macmillan.

Miller, L., Taylor, J., & Carver, M. H. (Eds.) (2003). *Voices made flesh: Performing women's autobiography*. Madison, Wisconsin: University of Wisconsin Press.

Miner, E. (1968). The traditions and forms of the Japanese poetic diary. *Pacific Coast Philology, 3*, 38–48. http://www.jstor.org/stable/1316671

More-Gilbert, B. (2009). *Postcolonial life-writing culture, politics and self-representation*. Abingdon, Oxon: Routledge.

Oakdale, S. (2005). *I foresee my life: The ritual performance of autobiography in an Amazonian community*. Lincoln and London: University of Nebraska Press.

Park-Fuller, L. (2003). A clean breast of it. In L. C. Miller, J. Taylor, & M. Carver (Eds.), *Performing women's autobiography: Voices made flesh* (pp. 215–236). Madison, Wisconsin: University of Wisconsin Press.

Pearlman, L. (2015). 'Dissemblage' and 'truth praps': Creating methodologies of resistance in queer autobiographical theatre. *Theatre Research International, 40*(1), 88–91.

Pendzik, S. (2013a). The poiesis and praxis of autobiographical therapeutic theatre. Keynote speech, *13th Summer Academy of the German Association of Theatre-Therapy* (DGFT), Remscheid, Germany. https://www.academia.edu/12635258/The_Poiesis_and_Praxis_of_Autobiographical_Therapeutic_Theatre

Pendzik, S. (2013b). The 6-Key Model and the assessment of the aesthetic dimension in dramatherapy. *Dramatherapy, 35*(2), 90–98.

Rycroft, C. (1983). *Psychoanalysis and beyond*. London: Chatto & Windus – Hogarth Press.

Sajnani, N. (2012). The implicated witness: Towards a relational aesthetic in dramatherapy. *Dramatherapy, 34*(1), 6–21.

Saldaña, J. (2003). Dramatizing data: A premier. *Qualitative Inquiry, 9*(2), 218–236.

Saldaña, J. (2011). *Ethnotheatre: Research from page to stage*. Walnut Creek, CA: Left Coast Press.

Sandhal, C. (2003). Queering the crip or creeping the queer? Intersections of queer and crip identities in solo autobiographical performances. *GLQ: A Journal of Lesbian and Gay Studies, 9*(1–2), 25–56.

Schechner, R. (2013). *Performance studies: An introduction* (3rd ed.). London: Routledge.

Schmor, J. B. (1994). Confessional performance: Postmodern culture in recent American theatre. *Journal of Dramatic Theory and Criticism, 9*(1), 157–172.

Smith, S., & Watson, J. (1998). Introduction: Situating subjectivity in autobiographical practices. In S. Smith & J. Watson (Eds.), *Women, autobiography, theory: A reader* (pp. 3–51). Madison, Wisconsin: The University of Wisconsin Press.

Smith, S., & Watson, J. (2010). *Reading autobiography: A guide for interpreting life narratives.* Minneapolis, MN: Minnesota University Press.

Snow, S., D'Amico, M., & Tanguay, D. (2003). Therapeutic theatre and well-being. *Arts in Psychotherapy, 30*(2), 73–82.

Spry, T. (2001). Performing autoethnography: An embodied methodological praxis. *Qualitative Inquiry, 7*(6), 706–732.

Spry, T. (2010). Call it swing: A jazz blues autoethnography. *Cultural Studies ↔ Critical Methodologies, 10*(4), 271–282.

Spry, T. (2011). *Body, paper, stage: Writing and performing autoethnography.* Walnut Creek, CA: Left Coast Press.

Stephenson, J. (2012). After the apple: Post-lapsarian realism in *Garden// Suburbia*—An autobiographical site-specific work. In R. Barker & K. Solga (Eds.), *New Canadian realisms: New essays on Canadian theatre volume 2* (pp. 68–86). Toronto: Playwrights Canada.

Thompson, J. (2009). Ah pava! Nathiye: Respecting silence and the performance of not-telling. In S. Jennings (Ed.), *Dramatherapy and social theatre: Necessary dialogues* (pp. 48–62). London: Routledge.

Walker, J. (1994). Reading genres across cultures: The example of autobiography. In L. Lawal (Ed.), *Reading world literature: Theory, history, practice* (pp. 203–236). Austin, TX: University of Texas Press.

Wallace, C. (2006). Monologue theatre, solo performance, and self as spectacle. In C. Wallace (Ed.), *Monologues: Theatre, performance, subjectivity* (pp. 1–16). Prague: Litteraria Pragensia.

Weber, A. (1990). *Teresa of Avila and the rhetoric of femininity.* Princeton: Princeton University Press.

PART I

Influences and Concepts

Influences of Experimental Theatre on the Emergence of Self-revelatory Performance

Stephen Snow

Phil Jones, in *The Arts Therapies: A Revolution in Healthcare* (Jones, 2005), makes a connection between development of the avant-garde in the arts and the emergence of the arts therapies. He points in particular to the creative explosion that took place at Black Mountain College in the early 1950s and, particularly, to the so-called '1st Happening' in 1952 that John Cage entitled *Theatre Piece No. 1*. Jones presents a description of this event, staged by Cage, with spontaneous dances by Merce Cunningham, in which performers improvised all over the space, and films and slides were projected on the walls (2005, p. 69). Perhaps his most significant statement in regards to this piece is: 'The people didn't play fictional characters, but were themselves' (2005, p. 69). I agree with Jones that this is a nodal point in the evolution of avant-garde and experimental theatre. It is a harbinger of what springs forth in the 1960s. It is the beginning of the demolition of the famous fourth wall of illusionistic theatre and a defining artistic moment for the implementation of the self in performance. Jones goes on to delineate the interface between theatre and

S. Snow, PhD, RDT-BCT (✉)
The Department of Creative Arts Therapies and Centre for the Arts in Human Development, Concordia University, Montreal, Quebec, Canada
e-mail: dramarx@sympatico.ca

© The Author(s) 2016
S. Pendzik et al. (eds.), *The Self in Performance*,
DOI 10.1057/978-1-137-53593-1_2

21

therapy that occurred within the Black Mountain College experiments: 'Actors and dramatists were adapting therapy-influenced techniques in their preparation, artists were making use of the ideas about consciousness to work with improvisation and discovery... such revolutions in the arts influenced the development of the arts therapies' (2005, p. 70).

This significant connection between experimental theatre and therapy is reiterated by Roose-Evans in his book, *Experimental Theatre: From Stanislavski to Today* (Roose-Evans, 1970). He describes how the work of the great experimental theatre director, Jerzy Grotowski, who will be cited many times in the following pages as a guide and inspiration to drama therapists, is really about using theatre as '... a means of "self-healing" in the Jungian sense' (p. 7). Finally, performance theorist and experimental theatre director Richard Schechner also suggests this deep connection between the avant-garde and therapy in his model for the *Efficacy/Entertainment Braid: Fifteenth to Twenty-First Centuries in English and American Theatre* (Schechner, 1977, p. 77). In the far upper right-hand corner of his diagram of this model, indicating the place where performance is the most immersed in the efficacy principle, he lists Avant-Garde and Psychodrama. Schechner writes: '... the avant-garde... by the mid-twentieth century, expanded to include direct political action, *psycho-therapy* (italics mine) and other manifestly efficacious kinds of performances' (1977, p. 78). It might be noted in regards to psychodrama, that its creator, Jacob Levy Moreno, had invented another form derived from it, and highly related to *self-revelatory performance* (Self-Rev), to which he gave the names autodrama or monodrama. Monodrama is a therapeutic format in which the client acts out all the persons in their life and all their interior projections, alone, by themselves. One famous therapist of the 1960s, Fritz Perls '... used monodrama as a core technique in Gestalt Therapy' (Blatner, 1973, p. 16). We can see in all of these various manifestations, from the experiments in performance at Black Mountain College in the 1950s to the influence of Grotowski's laboratory theatre in the 1960s, a genuine and organic interface between the developments in experimental theatre and parallel developments in the world of therapy, most significantly, the emergence of drama therapy.

Impact of Experimental Theatre on the Emergence of Drama Therapy

In many ways, drama therapy, as an emergent form of therapy, was incubated in the 1960s in the context of all the revolutions taking place in society and the arts. It was deeply impacted by this specific cultural period (Johnson &

Emunah, 2009; Jones, 1996). However, in examining the greatest theatrical influences on drama therapy, one has to go back to the earlier forms of experimental theatre and acknowledge that, in their own era, the work of Stanislavski and Brecht were immensely experimental (Roose-Evans, 1970). Prior to Grotowski, Stanislavski's articulation of *emotion memory* and Brecht's formulation of his *alienation effect,* were two major influences of theatre practice on the development of drama therapy methodology. Because of its interpretation, or misinterpretation, in the American *Method,* there is controversy around exactly what Stanislavski was proposing in his system of acting, including emotion memory (Benedetti in Stanislavski, 2008, p. xx). Regardless, it is certain that the great master acting teacher expected the actor to explore his or her own psychology and emotions. This is made very clear in the chapter on emotion memory in *An Actor Prepares:* '*You can never get away from yourself...* no matter how much you act, how many parts you take, you should never allow yourself any exception to the rule of using your own feelings' (Stanislavski, 1936, p. 167). This implies rigorous self-exploration and self-knowledge. No wonder this theory of acting is seen by Emunah to constitute an important influence on the development of drama therapy. This is equally true of Brecht's alienation effect; it sets the theoretical basis for Landy's foundational theory of distancing, which Landy expands upon: 'Brecht's theory of distancing is incomplete, as healthy functioning requires a balance of feeling and thought. A fuller understanding of distancing is that it is an interaction or intrapsychic phenomenon characterized by a range of closeness and separation' (Landy, 1986, p. 98). Elsewhere, Landy states that '... distancing is a central concept and tool in the dramatic treatment of clients and... the drama therapist can be more effective in his treatment if he can understand the dimensions of distancing...' (Landy, 1996, p. 14). Both Landy and Emunah acknowledge their debt to these earlier forms of experimental theatre which paved the way for the revolution in theatrical art in the 1960s and 1970s, and foreshadow the new way the self was to be represented in performance.

Landy (1982) recognizes the significant influence of Grotowski, Artaud and Julian Beck on the development of drama therapy theory. This same trio is cited by Emunah (1994) as having an immense effect upon the development of her own methods. Landy quotes how Grotowski saw his own method of actor training as kind of therapy: 'I am talking of the method, I am speaking of the surpassing of limits, of a confrontation, of a process of self-knowledge and, in a certain sense, of a therapy (Grotowski as quoted in Landy, 1982, p. 92). Many authors specifically cite Grotowski as a singular influence on their work, in particular Johnson (2009) regarding his method Developmental Transformations. Johnson and his colleagues' arti-cle, *Towards a Poor Drama Therapy*, in the *Arts and Psychotherapy* (Johnson, Forrester, Dintino, James, & Schnee, 1996) is probably the most completely articulated statement of the influence of a major voice of an experimental theatre practitioner on a single drama therapy method. As these authors point out: 'Grotowski's work shone a bright light on the path from theatre to therapy, which we have been traversing ever since' (1996, p. 295).

INFLUENCES OF EXPERIMENTAL THEATRE ON THE SELF-REVELATORY PERFORMANCE METHOD

In her seminal work on drama therapy, *Acting for Real: Drama Therapy Process, Technique and Performance* (1994), Emunah makes more than a dozen references to various experimental theatre practitioners who have influenced her thinking. She articulates this lucidly in the statement: 'Experimental theatre in the past several decades has paid increasing atten-tion to the process of acting, rather than focusing only on the product or performance. The ways in which various theatre directors and theorists have viewed acting and performance have had an important influence on the development of drama therapy' (1994, p. 8).

Emunah created the method of *self-revelatory performance* in 1983 (2014, p. 73). She has clearly defined this methodology and its development (Emunah, 1994, 2009, 2015), including in Chap. 3 of this volume. What is important here is how significant her understanding of the theories and practices of experimental theatre were to the creation of Self-Rev. In Chap. 10 of *Acting for Real*, she writes: 'Self-revelatory performance is not only a new kind of therapy, but a new genre of theatre. It builds upon the works of Grotowski, Artaud, the Living Theatre, and other experimental theatre directors and companies who explored boundaries, the actor's own process, and the relationship between the actor and audience' (1994, p. 291).

This is a portentous statement as it thrusts drama therapy into the domain of theatre—'a new genre of theatre'—with all the aesthetic con-siderations that this entails. In some ways, it even frames this performative form of drama therapy as a type of experimental theatre itself.

THE INFLUENCE OF ANTONIN ARTAUD

In many ways, Artaud became the poet-philosopher of the experimental theatre movement. His ideas were embodied most vividly in the work of *The Living Theatre*, one of the most radical theatre ensembles of the era.

Artaud was a complete rebel against the bourgeois theatre that he faced in France in the 1920s. One of his most famous sayings is: '... And if there is still one hellish, truly accursed thing in our time, it is our artistic dallying with forms, instead of being like *victims burnt at the stake, signaling through the flames*' (Artaud, 1958, p. 13; italics added). This latter phrase became the rallying cry of many radical theatre artists in the 1960s. Artaud, the madman, the poet, the visionary, urged the theatre artist to deep expressions of the psyche, outside the norms of naturalism and realism. He was really something of a mystic as well. His rhapsodic writing on the Balinese theatre, which he had experienced at the Paris Exposition in 1920, previewed the turn to the East, another element of the avant-garde theatre. On the other hand, Artaud could express concepts for the art of acting that were quite simple and graceful. My personal favorite is his Chaplinesque conception of actor as 'an athlete of the heart' (1958, p. 133). His ideas about *affective athleticism* were to have a great effect on acting styles in the 1960s and 1970s. Emunah cites the influence of Artaud on the development of Self-Rev: Artaud created an artistic theatre '... in which truths were revealed and emotional and spiritual purging occurred. Artaud used the language of dream, image, gesture, and poetry, breaking away from the theatre of his times, which was dominated by words and linear plot' (1994, p. 10). One can see in this quotation from Emunah's book, Artaud's brilliant and poetic thinking on theatre was having an influence on the development of a healing theatre.

THE INFLUENCE OF JERZY GROTOWSKI

Perhaps no one had a greater influence on the shift to the new conceptions of the art of acting than the Polish theatre director Jerzy Grotowski. In the words of Peter Brook: '... no one since Stanislavski has investigated the nature of acting, its phenomenon, its meaning, the nature and science of its mental-physical-emotional processes as deeply and completely as Grotowski' (Grotowski, 1969, p. 13). When Jerzy Grotowski swept into the American avant-garde theatre culture in the late 1960s, it was definitely as prophet of a whole new framework for acting. Within a few years, his notions of the *holy actor*, the *sacrum* of the theatre, and the *via negativa* had become common theatre parlance. His influence on experimental theatre director Richard Schechner was immense. Emunah relates how the concept of theatre presented by Grotowski and Artaud '... is not a way out (of our problems, pain, dilemmas, longings, etc.), but a profound journey inward. Acting with integrity, or being an audience to others who are acting with integrity, is a path toward deep knowing and healing' (1994, p. 11). So here we find the genuine interface between the theories of the art of acting emerging in the 1960s and the development of the Self-Rev. The powerful impact of Grotowski's concept of *self-penetration* is reiterated in the work of drama therapy students who undertake the Self-Rev as their final research project. One such student at Concordia University's Drama Therapy program used this Grotowski quote as emblematic of her work:

> 'If the actor, by setting himself a challenge publicly challenges others, and, through excess, profanation and outrageous sacrilege reveals himself by casting off his everyday mask, he makes it possible for the spectator to undertake a similar process of self penetration.' (Grotowski, as quoted in Furlong, 2010, p. 25)

THE LIVING THEATRE, OPEN THEATRE, AND THE PERFORMANCE GROUP

The third party mentioned by both Landy (1982) and Emunah (1994) as having influenced drama therapy is the Living Theatre. What exactly this influence on drama therapy was is somewhat difficult to pin down as the Living Theatre continually metamorphosed itself. Interestingly, its early history is very connected to two veterans of the Black Mountain College scene, Merce Cunningham and John Cage, who, in 1958, helped the Living Theatre find its Fourteenth Street theatre/rehearsal space. This company became the seedbed for the use of the personal self in performance. At the core, their mission was emancipation from political oppression—a kind of social therapy—which was deeply connected to psychological oppression. As Stefan Brecht writes about them:

> Though Artaud is kidding when he says his kind of theatre might purge civilization of its characteristic criminality, the Living Theatre, intending such a purge, has picked up on not only his stage tricks but his idea for content, *the misery & cruelty of civilization...* enacting something like the anarchist revolution. (1969, p. 52)

However, they were not only a radical political theatre, but were also psychologically radical as a performance group. The major goal of their work was to 'psychologistically attack *repression in the individual*—the original repression, self-repression, the source and origin of repression in society'

(Brecht, 1969, p. 48). They followed the psychosexual precepts of Wilhelm Reich and the radical social psychology of R.D. Laing. In fact, in *Paradise Now*, they chanted the last lines of Laing's book, *The Politics of Experience* (Laing, 1967): 'If I could turn you on, if I could drive you out of your wretched mind, if I could tell you I would let you know' (McDermott, 1969, p. 83). This was possibly the most extreme move towards the presentation of an authentic self in performance in the 1960s. The Laing quote epitomized a mantra of that era. It also articulated a *Weltanschauung* that saw the massive alienation of humanity, suffering from the horror of war after war, as the essential illness of culture to be cured. From Laing's view, so-called normality was itself a sickness. This manifested in the performance of *Paradise Now* by challenging every aspect of social repression (including the law against being naked in public), but also in a performance style that allowed for tremendous spontaneity and freedom of individual expression. As Julian Beck is quoted in relation to this performance: '...we have nothing except ourselves' (Schechner, 1969, p. 32). They used themselves to challenge the audience toward communal revolution, to 'open the doors to Paradise.' 'I am not allowed to take off my clothes!' the actors shout with hysterical frustration, hoping to catalyze spontaneous action by audience members.

The Living Theatre left an indelible mark on the culture of the 1960s. They had a Moreno-esque vision of a social therapy that like any 'truly therapeutic procedure cannot have less an objective than the whole of mankind' (Moreno, 1993, p. 3). Their revolution was, in this sense, like Laing's, a therapeutic revolution, freeing humankind from its 'mind-forged manacles.' As one critic wrote of the impact of their spectacles in 1968: 'The effect is immediately devastating and finally exhilarating, rather like a crash course in group therapy' (Secrest as quoted in Rostegno, 1970, p. 54).

The Open Theatre led by Joseph Chaikin and the Performance Group led by Richard Schechner were two other important experimental theatre groups at the time. Chaikin's work from the early 60s focused on the creative community of the ensemble (Blumenthal, 1977, p. 126). He 'urged actors to think of themselves as people who sometimes assumed theatrical roles, but otherwise were part of the community that included the audience as well as fellow performers' (Blumenthal, 1977, p. 118). Somewhat like Grotowski, he wanted the actor to remove the socially conditioned persona and be present to the audience with their core selves. As Blumenthal writes: 'Presence is the quality of being right here right now, with an awareness of the actual space and the actual moment and of the vital meeting of lives in that space and moment' (1977, p. 113). Chaikin's approach has had a great impact on acting training and furthered the move toward the actor developing a powerful personal presence in performance. Schechner, although perhaps best known for his development of environmental theatre (Schechner, 1973), was also highly influenced by Grotowski's approach to acting. In his extremely successful production of *Dionysus in 69* (Schechner, 1970), he began to experiment with the actors coming out of role and just presenting themselves. For instance, the actor who played Dionysus began by introducing him or herself as the god: 'My name is William Finley, son of William Finley... I've come here tonight...to announce my divinity...' (Schechner, 1970, p. 38). As the actor, Joan MacIntosh, who also played the character of Dionysus in the production, stated: 'The absurdity of telling 250 people that I am a god makes me laugh and the audience laughs with me and gradually the strength comes and the self-mockery fades away... My whole performance hinges on this scene' (Schechner, 1970, p. 48). In this seminal experimental theatre production, the presence of the personal self begins to emerge within the performance space.

THE SHIFT TOWARD THE PERSONAL SELF IN PERFORMANCE

To locate the emergence of personal self from behind the mask of character, we have to go back to the very beginnings of experimental theatre in America, in 1959. Arthur Sainer makes a brilliant analysis of what he calls the 'radical loosening of the fabric of drama [that] was taking place before our eyes' (1975, p. 12). He cites the Living Theatre's production of Jack Gelber's play, *The Connection*, in which during the performance, the actors switched '... between performers making character and performers being themselves... the performers were *in* themselves, comfortably in the context of self until those moments when Gelber's script called for them to take themselves out of self and back into the play...' (Sainer, 1975, p. 12). Sainer designates this as the nodal moment in American theatre when a new dramaturgy and new theory of performance evolved. Richard Schechner picks up on this radical loosening theme in his essay, 'Drama, Script, Theatre and Performance': 'My work in this area has been an attempt to make both performer and audiences aware of the overlapping but conceptually distinct realities of drama, script, theatre and performance' (1977, p. 44). This radical deconstruction of the performance frame becomes even more emphasized when he directs Spalding Gray in Sam Shepard's *The Tooth of Crime*.

The First Movements Towards Autoperformance: Spalding Gray

'Gray's use of himself as raw material represents a turning point in the history of acting no less significant than the innovations of Stanislavski and Brecht' (Lee Breuer as quoted in Copeland, *New York Times*, 3 June 1979). Schechner beautifully outlines the movement towards what he calls *autoperformance* (Schechner, 1982) in the work of Spalding Gray in his Foreword to Demastes' book, *Spalding Gray's America* (2008). The new genre is 'a one-person show, but in the more radical sense using the one person who is performing as the source of material being performed' (1982, p. 44). In TPG's 1970 production of *Commune* he had played himself as the 'character, Spalding,' but it is the time when Schechner directed him in *The Tooth of Crime* (1972–73) that marks the beginning of his journey into full autobiographical performance. Gray describes the process of being allowed to break out of character and be himself: 'It began to occur to me, What if I didn't rebuild my character? ... What might I say? And I think that's where the first curiosity and temptation came in that I might be able to publicly be Spalding Gray' (Gray as quoted in Schechner, 2008, p. xiv). Still, there was a next step. This was Gray's collaboration with director Elizabeth Lecompte in creating a piece on his mother's suicide, *Rumstick Road* (1977). According to the experimental theatre director Lee Breuer: 'With *Rumstick Road...* it's finally all out of the bag, the statement reads: I'm my own material on all fronts—visually, vocally, historically, spiritually, psychologically, intellectually, and emotionally. I am myself... [this]... is the *third new idea about acting in this century*' (italics mine) (Breuer as quoted in Copeland, 1979).

This is the beginning of the turn towards performing the personal self in theatre that was to have an immense influence in many domains, including drama therapy. It is what Hymes has designated as a *metaphrasis*, or an interpretive transformation of a genre (Ben-Amos & Goldstein, 1975, p. 20). *Rumstick Road* is the transitional moment leading to this transformation. After *Rumstick Road*, Gray began a series of autobiographical pieces. These commenced with *Sex and Death to the Age 14* (1979) and culminated in *Swimming to Cambodia* (1985), which was later made into a commercial film by Jonathan Demme. In *Rumstick Road*, Gray had theatrically presented some of his most painful personal material in public. It was a relatively easy step, then, to go onstage, by himself, and tell stories about his personal life. As Schechner cites: '... the progression of Gray is particularly complete: a model of the move from actor-as-interpreter through performer in environmental theatre to autoperformer' (1982, p. 45).

Other performers in American Theatre were highly influenced by Gray's innovations. As Young records: 'Los Angeles-based director Mark W. Travis, who witnessed *Cambodia* in its stage incarnation, has since functioned as midwife for three successful one-man shows of an autobiographical nature' (1989, p. 179). At least two of these dealt with serious psychological issues that challenged the performers. The first, Paul Linke's solo piece, *Time Flies When You're Alive*, was about the performer's loss of his wife to breast cancer and the effect of this event on both himself and his family. Spalding Gray saw it and said that it was: '… the most vivid and intense solo theatre I have ever seen… a fine balance between a life lived and a life reflected upon' (Young, 1989, p. 183). The second piece, developed and performed by actor Shane McCabe, dealt with the personally devastating effects of childhood abuse. As with Gray's autoperformance pieces on highly intimate personal material, audience members came up to the actor after his performance of *No Place Like Home* and shared their personal experiences with him (Young, 1989, p. 185).

The 1987 National Association for Drama Therapy 8th Annual Conference, held at NYU, had as its theme: 'Performance and Healing in Drama Therapy.' It was in the air—all the connections of acting and healing. Renée Emunah, who had not yet published her seminal book, *Acting for Real* (1994), gave a three-hour workshop on 'Creating Self-Revelatory Performance.' The conference opened with an 'autobiographical healing piece,' *America's Finest*, by the professional actor Burke Byrnes. It dealt with the traumas of his childhood and adulthood in regards to learning to be a man. Burke had gone to see Spalding's monologue, *47 Beds*, and was very impressed with Spalding's ability to be so open about homosexuality and to freely, and in public, question his masculinity. Burke said that this inspired him to be able to be open about such taboo areas in his own life.

COMPARING AUTOBIOGRAPHICAL AND SELF-REV PERFORMANCES

The power of telling private truths in a public space seems to be one of the most dynamic components of both autoperformance and Self-Rev. What is the difference between Burke Brynes' piece, a Spalding Gray autoperformance and an Emunah-influenced Self-Rev? Emunah's position is that in the Self-Rev the psychological and emotional issues are really getting *worked through*, rather than merely presented, and this implies an effective therapy process that coincides with the acting process. I concur with this assessment. However, Emunah goes further by stating that there are differences in the levels of emotional intensity between these forms:

> *Self-Revelatory Performance* is distinguished from autobiographical the-atre in that in addition to being based on one's real life, it presents issues whose exposure demands a high level of risk-taking, partly because they are current issues, rather than past issues which have already been resolved. Autobiographical theatre, for example, can involve storytelling about past adventures (a la Spalding Gray) without being intensively intimate or emo-tionally on-the-line, whereas *Self-Revelatory Performance* is always on the emotional edge. (1994, p. 224)

In my view, Gray's earliest works, such as the transitional piece, *Rumstick Road*, have great emotional authenticity and intensity. *New York Times* theatre critic Richard Eder wrote of *Rumstick Road*: '... a brilliant and engrossing work; one whose abstraction and complexity are at the service of genuine emotion' (Jacket of *Rumstick Road*, Video Reconstruction, Wooster Group, 2013). Indeed, many autobiographical performances carry strong emotional valency, reflecting the talents of effective acting, which also requires high levels of emotional risk-taking.

Yet, despite the power of his work, did Spalding Gray have a therapeutic intention and/or experience from his developing and performing auto-biographical theatre? Was his deeply self-revelatory performance art heal-ing for himself, personally? After *Rumstick Road*, which could be called a genuinely self-revelatory piece, he began to move towards the solo pieces. These were minimalist person-to-person 'narratives of self-presentation' (Schechner, 1982, p. 47) in which he sat behind a table with a bottle of water, a notebook and a tape-recorder and told personal experiences from his life, as in *Sex and Death up to the Age of Fourteen, Booze, Cars and College Girls*, and *Forty-Seven Beds*. There is no evidence in any of this work that the performer had a conscious intention for the performance to be therapeutic. Working with the theme of his mother's suicide, as in *Rumstick Road*, he may have been attempting to come to terms with this traumatic event, but probably not a conscious working through in the therapeutic meaning of that term. As Demastes states: 'From major events like his mom's suicide to minor happenings throughout his life, by giving them order, he gives himself the opportunity to tolerate the memories he can't escape. That's how Gray's art saved him from a life of overwhelmingly consuming regret' (Demastes, 2008, p. 208). Watching the new video reconstruction of the performance of *Rumstick Road* (2013), one feels the sincerity of Gray's presence, the truthfulness of his telling, the genuine emotion evoked by the art and craft of experimental theatre explored by his director and his fellow actors. '*RR* has the grace—and I use this word knowingly—of redeeming the invasion of privacy by putting it in the service of a performer's attempt to comprehend two lives: those of Elizabeth Horton Gray and her son, Spalding Gray' (Schechner, 1982, p. 47). However, he never labeled it as being a healing piece as Burke Brynes had with his own solo piece.

Spalding Gray kept his art and his therapy in separate domains. In 1975, while traveling in India with the Performance Group, he had a nervous breakdown and, once back in New York, he sought the help of a psychiatrist (Casey, 2012, pp. 43–4). Interestingly, it was not long after this that he went to work on *Rumstick Road*. Because of all the resonances of mental illness, psychiatry and therapy surrounding it, I think this piece probably comes the closest to be a Self-Rev in Emunah's sense of this terminology. But it stops short, as Gray's concerns were more about art than using the theatre as a form of self-therapy. He was a very gifted performer and, over the course of the next decade, he developed his own unique style of autobiographical monologue. His entertainment potential became so great with these solo pieces that Mel Gussow of the *New York Times* could go so far as to call him a '"sit-down monologuist with the comic sensibility of a stand-up comedian"' (Gussow as quoted in Casey, 2012, p. 102). Nowhere is this capacity to entertain and to artfully tell stories more apparent than in the Jonathan Demme Hollywood release of *Swimming to Cambodia* (1987). Gray is absolutely mesmerizing in this film version of his famous monologue. One sees a mature artist at work, weaving together, with consummate skill, the magic of his words, his images and his performance.

Spalding Gray made his life into art: he was a courageous, risk-taking artist. Although he kept his therapy and theatre separate, he often plunged into the heart of darkness by 'mining my own psychic landscapes' (Gray as quoted in Young, 1989, p. 178). He was a pioneer in the theatre who showed a way for others to explore personal issues via the art of theatre, though sadly in the end it seemed he was unable to resolve his personal psychological issues through his art or indeed by other means.

CONCLUSION

There have been many influences on drama therapy theorists and practitioners from the experimental theatre movement. Many of the leading scholars in drama therapy cite the powerful impact on their thinking of figures like Artaud, Grotowski and the Living Theatre. Some go so far as to say that one figure has been the primary source of their own methodology (Johnson, 2009; Johnson et al., 1996). The originator of the Self-Rev method has pointed to the dynamic influence of Grotowski on her development of this methodology, especially his concept of self-penetration as an acting method (Emunah, 1994, p. 10). In a holistic way, the innovative autoperformance work of Spalding Gray—which Breuer (in Copeland, 1979) called the 'the third new idea about acting in this century'—has also helped to shape the conceptualization of Self-Rev. In this sense, the Self-Rev is itself a new genre of experimental theatre.

Emunah makes a substantial case for her method as serving both a therapeutic and an aesthetic function. She writes: 'Some people hold that if art is intentionally therapeutic it cannot be truly art, but Self-Rev breaks that myth. Self-Rev manages to hold the tension between art and therapy. Neither component is sacrificed; rather, both are amplified' (Emunah, 2015, p. 81). It is an exciting and challenging idea. This coincidence of art and healing is essential to the Self-Rev. It goes far beyond the concept that 'Theatre is therapy if a performance improves the psychological health of the spectators' (Kirby, 1976, p. 3). What differentiates it more than anything else from other forms of autobiographical theatre is the challenge of consciously working on a significant psychological issue that contemporaneously disturbs the life of the performer. As Emunah writes: 'The working through aspect of the Self-Revs leave performers with a sense of mastery and a new state of mind/heart, rather than with the unsettled raw vulnerability that could come from disclosure only' (2015, p. 78). This points to a paradigmatic differentiation that Phil Jones makes between theatre process and the drama therapy process: 'The chief difference between theatre and Dramatherapy here is that the Dramatherapy experience allows for the exploration and resolution of projections whereas the theatre only invites an expression of projected feelings' (Jones, 1996, p. 135).

Self-revelatory performance, deeply rooted in experimental and avant-garde theatre, and nourished by the insights and therapeutic orientation of the field of drama therapy, seems ready to be recognized as a new form of therapeutic theatre, inaugurated by the publication of this book.

REFERENCES

Artaud, A. (1958). *The theater and its double* (M. C. Richards, Trans.). New York: Grove Press.

Ben-Amos, D., & Goldstein, K. S. (Eds.) (1975). *Folklore: Performance and communication*. Paris: Mouton & Co.

Blatner, A. (1973). *Acting-in: Practical applications of psychodramatic methods*. New York: Springer.

Blumenthal, E. (1977). Joseph Chaikin: An open theory of acting. *Yale/Theatre*, *8*(2&3), 112–133.

Brecht, S. (1969). Revolution at the Brooklyn Academy of Music. *The Drama Review*, *13*(3), 47–73.

Casey, N. (Ed.) (2012). *The journals of spalding gray*. New York: Vintage Books.

Copeland, R. (1979, June 3). New York: *New York Times*, Arts and Leisure Section.

Emunah, R. (1994). *Acting for real: Drama therapy process, technique, and performance*. New York: Brunner-Mazel; Taylor and Francis.

Emunah, R. (2009). The integrative five phase model of drama therapy. In D. Johnson & R. Emunah (Eds.), *Current approaches in drama therapy* (pp. 37–64). Springfield, IL: C. C. Thomas.

Emunah, R. (2015). Self-revelatory performance: A form of drama therapy and theatre. *Drama Therapy Review*, *1*(1), 71–85.

Furlong, J. (2010). Exploring the hero's journey as a transformative experience: Self-revelatory performance as personal therapy and healing (Unpublished Master's research paper). Concordia University, Montreal.

Grotowski, J. (1969). *Towards a poor theatre*. New York: Simon and Schuster.

Johnson, D. R. (2009). Developmental transformations: Towards the body as presence. In R. Emunah & D. R. Johnson (Eds.), *Current approaches in drama therapy* (pp. 89–116). Springfield, IL: C. C. Thomas.

Johnson, D., & Emunah, R. (Eds.) (2009). *Current approaches in drama therapy*. Springfield, IL: C.C. Thomas.

Johnson, D. R., Forrester, A., Dintino, C., James, M., & Schnee, G. (1996). Towards a poor drama therapy. *Arts in Psychotherapy*, *23*(4), 293–306.

Jones, P. (1996). *Drama as therapy, theatre as living*. London: Routledge.

Jones, P. (2005). *The arts therapies: A revolution in healthcare*. New York: Brunner-Routledge.

Kirby, M. (1976). Introduction to the theatre and therapy issue. *The Drama Review*, *20*(1), 3.

Laing, R. D. (1967). *The politics of experience and the bird of paradise*. Harmondsworth, Middlesex. England: Penguin Books.

Landy, R. (1982). Training the drama therapist—A four-part model. *Arts in Psychotherapy*, *9*, 91–99.

Landy, R. (1986). *Drama therapy: Concepts and practices.* Springfield, IL: C. C. Thomas.

Landy, R. (1996). *Essays in drama therapy: The double life.* London: Jessica Kinsley.

McDermott, P. (1969). Portrait of an actor, watching: Antiphonal feedback to the Living Theatre. *The Drama Review, 13*(3), 74–83.

Moreno, J. L. (1993). *Who shall survive: Foundations of sociometry, group psychotherapy and sociodrama* (student ed.). McLean, VA: American Society for Group Psychotherapy and Psychodrama.

Roose-Evans, J. (1970). *Experimental theatre: From Stanislavski to today.* New York: Routledge.

Rostegno, A. (1970). *We, the living theatre.* New York: Ballantine Books, Inc..

Sainer, A. (1975). *The radical theatre notebook.* New York: Avon.

Schechner, R. (1969). Containment is the enemy: Judith Malina and Julian Beck interviewed by Richard Schechner. *The Drama Review, 13*(3), 24–46.

Schechner, R. (Ed.). (1970). *Dionysus in 69: The performance group.* New York: Farrar, Straus and Giroux.

Schechner, R. (1973). *Environmental theatre.* New York: Hawthorne Books.

Schechner, R. (1977). *Essays in performance theory, 1970–1977.* New York: Drama Book Specialists.

Schechner, R. (1982). *The end of humanism: Writings on performance.* New York: Performing Arts Journal Publications.

Schechner, R. (2008). Foreword: Spalding. In W. W. Demastes (Ed.), *Spalding Gray's America* (pp. ix–xxi). New York: Limelight Editions.

Stanislavski, C. (1936). *An actor prepares* (E. R. Hapgood, Trans.). New York: Theatre Arts Books.

Stanislavski, C. (2008). *An actor's work: A student's diary* (J. Benedetti, Ed. and Trans.). London: Routledge.

The Wooster Group (Producer). (2013). *Video reconstruction of Rumstick Road by Ken Kobland and Elizabeth Lecompte with Clay Hapaz, Matt Schloss and Max Bernstein* [DVD]. Available from www.thewoostergroup.org

Young, J. R. (1989). *Acting solo: The art of one-man shows.* Beverly Hill, CA: Moonstone Press.

CHAPTER 3

From Behind the Scenes to Facing an Audience in Self-Revelatory Performance

Renée Emunah

Self-revelatory performance, a form of drama therapy and theatre, involves the creation of an original theatrical piece based on current personal issues in need of investigation, healing or transformation. The development of self-revelatory performance (Self-Rev), and its relationship to autobiographical and therapeutic theatre, have been described in a recent article, 'Self-Revelatory Performance: A Form of Drama Therapy and Theatre' (Emunah, 2015). That article focuses on the theatrical *working through* of personal material—an essential component of Self-Revs, including methods of dramatically grappling with and therapeutically healing struggles, at the same time ensuring the development of a work of art worthy of presentation before an audience. This chapter takes a close look at the journey leading up to the performance of a Self-Rev. The intensive exploratory process involving a creative collaboration between performer and director is examined. As the Self-Rev process culminates in a live performance, the interaction with an audience, along with the role the audience plays in such intimate theatrical productions, are explored. The potential pitfall in Self-Rev of self-indulgence is then addressed, along with articulating the ways in which the personal translates into the universal, and sociocultural dimensions intersect with the personal.

R. Emunah, PhD, RDT-BCT (✉)
Drama Therapy Graduate Program, California Institute of Integral Studies, San Francisco, CA, USA
e-mail: remunah@ciis.edu

© The Author(s) 2016   37
S. Pendzik et al. (eds.), *The Self in Performance,*
DOI 10.1057/978-1-137-53593-1_3

THE PERFORMER'S AND THE DIRECTOR'S PROCESS

EARLY STAGES

Performer and director straddle the thin line between constructing a personal healing process and creating a final product that speaks to an audience. There is a gradual progression from the former to the latter, though both are always at play.

Self-Rev performers ideally possess a background in theatre performance and a capacity for psychological introspection. With these combined interests, it is not surprising that many are drama therapists. Self-Rev performances have been used in drama therapy training, including as a capstone project (Emunah, Raucher, & Ramirez, 2014), and in clinical and theatrical arenas. Directors are typically registered drama therapists, with strong directing and clinical skills.

In the early stages of the process of creating a Self-Rev, performer and director mine inner landscapes, as they search for what is most essential to explore. Sometimes a performer is clear from the outset about the issue/s to be tackled. But generally, many matters emerge, and the initial work entails deciphering what has the most 'heat,' that is, which issues feel most current, charged, in process, and significant or even urgent to the performer. This early exploration parallels what happens in therapy sessions: In a single therapy hour, once a week, not everything can be explored, and a skillful therapist helps steer the conversation toward the more germane themes. A client may begin talking about one matter that is indirectly linked to a more salient issue. Similarly, in the early Self-Rev process, performer and director aim to get closer to what is most authentic and relevant. While in most cases there is a sense of having too many issues and the process involves distillation, some performers have the opposite challenge: they are not sure whether they have any issues of sufficient significance. It could be that they are not ripe to work on a Self-Rev, though in most cases issues of surprising significance do emerge.

'Issues' is used for lack of a better word, as typically Self-Revs revolve around core and ongoing life themes and struggles, or events or aspects of one's life that have had profound implications. How is this current? The matter/s have now come to the forefront of the performer's awareness and s/he is ready to place them at center stage—spotlighting the ways in which these themes impact the present—and potentially the future. The performer has a need/desire to grapple with and bring healing to these matters. This healing may lead to a kind of closure, and/or to an opening—of what lies ahead.

While some directors utilize primarily verbal modes to help performers elicit or clarify salient themes, most work in-action, incorporating drama therapy methods along with a variety of theatre and movement-based processes to invite paramount issues to the surface. Regardless of the methods used in these early stages, directors are attentive to developing trust with the performer, and encouraging the performer's strengths, vulnerability, authenticity, and freedom of expression.

The director will be the performer's first audience. One performer wrote (in her journal, post-performance):

> The places I had been hurt in my life had occurred in relationship. I longed for more connection and for the freedom that comes from knowing oneself in the presence of another. As the parallel process between my original trauma and the self-rev process became clear to me, I noticed how fearful I felt that my process would not be respected by my director. (But) my director accepted me unconditionally... and held my grief and emotions with compassion and care. This was exactly what I needed early in the process... to be able to fully invest myself and reveal more of myself... (Dorothy Lemoult, 2011)

Performers work on their own as well—writing, journaling, reflecting on their dreams, dramatizing, painting, dancing, and noticing themselves in action. There can be a surge of both creativity and self-observation. Present-day life experiences often generate heightened scrutiny and fresh discovery. Everything that happens becomes potential grist for the developing performance piece.

Once the subject matter of the Self-Rev is clear, the heart of the work begins—which entails diving into this material, examining it from multiple angles, and broadening the scope of exploration—often in unexpected ways. At the same time that new associations to the issue/s are uncovered, director and performer ensure that the process (and ultimately product) do not become merely unprocessed autobiography, but rather stay on the path of deepening the understanding and healing of the struggle/s. The multidimensional and intensive exploratory process between performer and director ultimately leads to burrowing into the matters of greatest centrality, albeit ones that may have been buried or denied until this point in time.

Later Stages

As the overall narrative of the piece is clarified, performer and director examine autobiographical components, ascertaining what information is central to the understanding of the piece. Performer and director explore how to communicate these components succinctly, often consolidating factual personal information in creative ways. One performer, Daniel Smith, in *Root* (2012), depicted the constant relocations in his childhood by a frantic moving about the stage. A silent character on the side of the stage stood by a blackboard that had a list of all the locations Daniel had lived in; each time another move was referred to, the character simply crossed off that location. The simplicity of this gesture, combined with Daniel's corresponding tearing off a piece of his cloth garment, was poignant and concise, and meant that little background storytelling was needed.

Questions about disclosure will arise: What is essential to tell, what is the performer un/comfortable disclosing, what is beyond the scope of this piece? Additionally, there are often psychological or ethical concerns related to implicating other real people in one's piece. Carolyn Ellis (2007), referring to the related field of autoethnographic and personal narrative research, suggests a 'relational ethics of care' (reminiscent of Nisha Sajnani's *relational aesthetics* in drama therapy, 2012). In referring to Ellis' work and to autoethnographic writing and performance, Poulous discusses the dilemma: 'These stories cannot be told, but they cannot not be told!... What might this... falling out of secret, crafted into story, do to or for those whose stories I tell?' (2009, p. 130).

There are many other—both aesthetic and therapeutic—considerations, such as whether to perform solo or include auxiliary actors, and determining theatrical styles that bring out the performer's strengths and best elucidate particular issues.

Each and every phase and question is challenging. Yet the greatest challenge is at the very core of Self-Rev: how one authentically works through and begins to heal the presented issues. How do the performer and director reach deeply enough into the heart and soul of the issues being grappled with to gradually, in steps and layers, achieve change, healing, or transformation? This process takes time, along with willingness on the part of the performer and clinical skills on the part of the director. The question of what constitutes healing will emerge for both director and performer.

What does 'working through' mean? It means that there is a conscious effort to contend with the material, dive into it, untangle the issues and better comprehend their origins and implications. It means psychological self-examination as well as ownership of our own interplay with the forces that shaped us. And it means finding ways to be strengthened or softened or altered by the material, and to 'move through it.' What does moving through mean? It can mean letting go, taking hold of, coming to terms with, confronting, embracing, shifting, admitting, committing, forgiving, inviting, renewing, revolting, revisiting, recreating. Each individual and each issue is different, with particular features and complexities, so there are no formulas. (Emunah, 2015, pp. 74–5)

One performer reflected:

The awareness of my personal process paralleling the aesthetic realm was a consistent, measurable guide to me throughout. One of the most interesting things was to observe how much easier it was for me to reveal some of the secret things that I am currently struggling with than for me to reveal and explore what was behind and what lies underneath all these issues— which is precisely why this process is therapeutic. (Jesse Jo Toth, 2011)

Resistance may well emerge as one confronts internal barriers, social pressures, fears, homeostasis, and ingrained patterns. However, one's particular forms of resistance can lead not only to further insight but can also be used theatrically. Many performers dramatically depict their resistance within their performance pieces. In her piece, entitled *Inner World Lullabies*, Jesse Jo Toth (2011) embodied her 'inner critic,' along with two other internal characters—a gung-ho 'mental health cheerleader' and her 'true self.' Through these characters she explored her various vices; her fears about love, life, and being a therapist; and her resistance to self-examination (which created an interesting paradox, as here she was performing a Self-Rev!). Another performer, Elyssa Kilman, in *This is about Heartbreak* (2009), embodied a Protector/Jewish Mother, who tried to talk her out of becoming vulnerable and even of doing the Self-Rev piece. Performer Jenelle Mazaris, in her piece *Little Miss Self* (2008), played with her fear of going out onto the stage, keeping the audience waiting. Finally a tough inner protector character emerged (with boxing gloves!) explaining to the audience that Jenelle would not be doing the piece. Then a 'gossip girl' character entered, confiding to the audience secrets about Jenelle. As Jenelle herself had supposedly not shown up for the piece, a crisis management team began to search for her.

The theatrical playing out of resistance—a kind of acting out but with the deliberate consciousness of acting (Blatner, 1988; Emunah, 1994, 1995)—typically adds both humor and pathos to a piece, and eases the way for performers to plow past these resistances into uncharted personal terrain.

Performer and director note lines and moments occurring spontaneously during the improvisational and drama therapeutic workshop processes that are striking, powerful, poignant, evocative, enlightening, clarifying, humorous, or significant. Also recorded are therapeutic methods and moments that are theatrically compelling. Ultimately, the material needs to be shaped and a script created—out of the raw stuff that emerges in the process.

A script is gradually drafted. But because Self-Rev is based on what is current, the script constantly evolves. Real-life occurrences during the course of preparing a Self-Rev may impact the piece. One performer was creating a piece about his fear of being alone, and during the process/rehearsal period he began a new and promising relationship—which certainly had a bearing on the piece (and perhaps vice versa!). The piece grows alongside the person's life, and the person's life is influenced by the work on the piece.

The focus for performer and director shifts to honing, chiseling, and editing the script. There may be bits that are extraneous or distracting to the essence of the piece, and other segments that warrant elaboration. Some lines may require greater clarity or succinctness. The director's job shifts from being process-oriented to refining the product; at this point her work is more in keeping with traditional directing, including enhancing the actor's skills, and fine-tuning details such as gesture, intonation, expression, and stage movement. Music, sound, stage set, lighting, and props are considered. The director is actively engaged in holding, shaping, and perfecting the overall production. Often both performer and director have new sparks of creativity during this period, adding elements that embellish the show. The actor is also working on memorizing and rehearsing the script.

The ending moment of the piece is of critical importance and often goes through many reiterations and may not be discovered or finalized until late in the rehearsal process. Certain questions need to be considered: What does the performer want to leave the audience with? What does she want to leave herself with? Does the ending encapsulate or punctuate the piece, in a way that is aesthetic, potent and clear? Does it avoid simplistic or pat resolutions? Does it enhance the power or poignancy of the piece? And unlike these last few sentences, strong endings generally do not close with question marks!

As the performance date nears and the reality of an audience becomes more palpable, the performer often experiences new fears. The director should have a strong and calming presence at this point, helping the performer navigate these concerns. Drama therapy methods are conducive to addressing anxieties, and preparing the performer for feelings that may emerge the night of the performance and afterwards. Generally, as the performance date approaches, anxiety turns into excitement, and the performer feels a readiness to release the piece to an audience.

The Self-Rev Performer and the Audience

The process leading up to the moment of sharing the piece before an audience has been a gradual and relational one, between performer and director, along with the performer's singular excavation of inner pain, discovery of resources and resilience, and unraveling layers of insight. A new element, which continues the journey of externalization and bringing to light what may have been dormant, is now being introduced: sharing the production with an audience. Performers need to ready themselves for this momentous encounter.

All actors warm up before performances, yet the warm-ups immediately before a Self-Rev are vital. They should address both theatrical and personal aspects of a Self-Rev. Voice and body are energized; the performer prepares to be fully present on stage. But this presence on stage is not one of persona, but of person, the performer as her truest self. And not just self, but self about to change, in the presence of an audience. The warm-up techniques should facilitate an openness to being in deep connection with the audience and with oneself. The performer is not only about to make an offering to an audience, but is about to receive a formidable gift: a culmination, intensification, and solidification of the healing in the Self-Rev process. The warm-ups need to create a readiness to receive this gift, along with a capacity to feel the emotions that come with it.

The warm-ups ideally invigorate all parts of the performer's being, her many selves, including her bravery; indeed, a boldness is needed to perform a Self-Rev, a strength that invites and contains vulnerability. The quality of warm-up preparation right before the show can affect the performer's presence and the balance of emotional distancing in the piece.

The performer needs to show up for the audience and for herself. Many performers become tearful during this warm-up, as they are suddenly struck by the personal significance of what is about to transpire. One warm-up that is unique to Self-Rev is to have the performer stand in the center of a circle of peers (auxiliary actors or people that have directly supported the theatrical process). She then states various words of affirmation or reminders that would be helpful to hear. As the performer gently falls and is held within the circle, the surrounding people repeat these overlapping phrases, in their own manners.

The content of the performance piece often strikes the performer in new ways (cognitively, emotionally, and spiritually) as she shares it with an audience. While all performance involves an actor's vulnerability and relationship with an audience, the therapeutic change occurring within Self-Revs takes this vulnerability and connection with an audience to new levels. Much is at stake. While all theatre is transitory in nature, many Self-Rev theatre pieces are performed only once, before a single audience, highlighting the ephemeral nature of performance and yet at the same time heightening a sense of ritual or rite of passage, in which something of long-range repercussion is being marked and imprinted.

Performer Marissa Snoddy (2011) reflected:

> Before going on stage, my biggest worries were getting my lines and how much time it (the performance piece) would take. Once I got into (the character of) Mama Fire, it felt like I was just riding a wave. I felt like I was living my piece, not just acting in it. It all felt very present for me.

Many performers have noticed that particular lines or segments within their piece elicit new levels of insight or unanticipated emotionality while on stage. The audience's witnessing affects the performer's connection to the content of the piece, and amplifies realizations. The palpable connection between audience and performer reinforces the significance of acts of healing or transformation, further layering the therapeutic impact. One performer created an intense piece revolving around childhood sexual abuse. At one point she faced the audience, softly stating, as though for the first time, 'I'm a survivor.' The audience, who had been in a state of hushed silence for some time, suddenly broke into a loud and prolonged applause. At that unexpected moment, the performer registered this simple line more deeply, receiving the audience's unflinching recognition of her.

When the piece ends, and the audience applauds (often as a standing ovation), it is recommended that the performer breathe, take in the audience's response, and remain present. Following the applause, performers normally spend quiet moments alone or with their director (or close friend). Digesting the experience is important, and will come in stages, but the moments right after the show are precious. There has been a kind of birth.

Self-Rev performers typically experience not only surges of relief and accomplishment, but also waves of self-acceptance and the churning of change being activated. There is much to digest, and it is recommended that directors and performers meet at least twice after the performance, to fuse process and product, achieve closure, and prepare for post-performance stages. Naturally, psychological healing, along with life's continued unfolding, is an ongoing process. The Self-Rev, while signifying a huge milestone and representing accelerated therapeutic growth and creative mastery, is nonetheless not a panacea. There can be some unrest, as one assimilates the intense internal changes that have taken place through the Self-Rev process and performance. Directors can help performers integrate new growth, celebrate achievement, and stay attuned to the next chapter of their journeys.

Over the past decade, I have found that there seems to be less *post-performance depression* or letdown following Self-Revs than after other forms of therapeutic theatre performances (Emunah, 1994; Emunah & Johnson, 1983). This may be linked to the degree and depth of healing within Self-Revs (and therefore there is variance between Self-Revs as well). Performances that emphasize disclosure but do not fully work on therapeutic levels leave performers much more unsettled and prone to post-performance depression than pieces that are solidly rooted as quality healing Self-Revs. For example, if a Self-Rev piece revolves around experiences of trauma without including a depth of healing, or recounts injustices or grievances without self-examination, there may be an unconscious hope of being taken care of, overtly validated, or even rescued by the audience, which leads ultimately to disappointment. Performers whose pieces are heavily disclosing but therapeutically static are likely to feel more unresolved or overly exposed afterwards. Obviously pat resolutions or aspirational endings in theatre pieces that have not entailed a depth and multiplicity of healing methods leave a superficial and short-lived sense of victory, which could well be followed by a period of distress. As Self-Revs' primary ingredient is an honest attempt at healing, via drama therapy methods, the above caveats are important.

An intriguing factor is that after some therapeutic theatre performances, participant-performers feel that the capacities they manifested in their performances far exceeded their capacities in real life. This gap, along with the 'return to reality' or to their 'former selves,' can be disconcerting and painful. In Self-Rev, there is less of a gap. The performer is reaching for something—healing and hope—but the entire process/product is so real and has involved so much working through that afterwards the person typically feels enveloped in a state of acceptance, grace, and gratitude, rather than a sense of having to catch up with what was exhibited. There is also the sheer relief of sharing oneself, one's story, and one's discoveries with others.

A week after her Self-Rev (*The Buzzing Broken Beat of Life*, 2011), Marissa Snoddy wrote:

> Post-Self-Rev, I've felt many things. There are moments where I feel like I'm floating on a cloud. I feel a greater responsibility to my self and my emotions. I feel very open and intuitive. Translating my story into a theatrical piece felt incredibly empowering. I felt myself claiming my story for myself, which also shifted my relationship to my story. I feel lighter because I'm not carrying it all alone. There are other people in this world who are holding the story with me.

Performer Dorothy Lemoult (*Mal de Mer*, 2011) wrote:

> I felt authentic and connected in ways I never had performing other theatre pieces. I saw that I had turned my separateness into togetherness, my pain into understanding, my suffering into hope. This is what I have always known theatre and therapy could do.

THE ROLE OF THE AUDIENCE

In a survey conducted of alumni of the CIIS Drama Therapy Program who had performed a capstone Self-Rev, the facet of the Self-Rev process rated the most effective (by our 43 respondents) in terms of healing (out of 15 given facets/factors) was 'performing the piece before an audience of empathic witnesses' (Emunah et al., 2014, p. 114).

Most audiences are seeing Self-Revs for the first time, and do not know what to expect, or if anything is expected of them. Audience members should receive a tad of introductory information, but without burdening them or setting any particular expectations. Simply telling audience members that Self-Revs are intimate theatre pieces exploring and healing personal struggles—and that their role is to watch what is about to take place with an open heart—suffices. The audience will indeed be entertained by compelling theatre, but there is a shift from its more common role of receptive viewer to that of empathic witness. The audience will soon realize that it is subtly implicated in the actor's healing, an awareness that heightens engagement and presence.

The invitation to the audience to witness the piece with an open heart is not only for the actor but also for the audience, as it is likely that the piece will touch audience members in personal and emotional ways. However, the audience should not feel encumbered by the actor's struggles. The actor may be unleashing a burden, but he is also owning this burden. In a strong Self-Rev, the audience feels deeply moved by the performer but does not feel the weight of taking care of the performer, nor fearful after the show for the performer's well-being. Audience members who know the performer intimately may be particularly stirred, with feelings of empathy, care, love, and awe for the person on stage. Yet the audience should not feel the need to let go of its critical mind in connecting to the performer and the piece. 'The audience's identification with the performer and natural inclinations to "root" for him/her need to be balanced by the performer's capacity to therapeutically master the presented issues and artistically master the piece. Without this therapeutic and artistic mastery, the audience could bear unnecessary concern or even pity for the actor and feel weighted down rather than fulfilled by the piece' (Emunah, 2015, p. 79).

In introducing Self-Rev, it is helpful to gently inform the audience that the performer may be in a tender, even altered, state following the performance. Such pre-empting helps audience members to be sensitive in their interactions with performers after the piece. In contrast, autobiographical performances often encourage post-performance dialogue, mingling, and interaction between performer and audience. After a Self-Rev, however, the performer is in a much more vulnerable state, as a live healing has just taken place and is still being integrated. Audiences too, following a Self-Rev, can be in a tender place, given all that may be stirred in their own psyches—not only in relation to the particular content of the Self-Rev but simply by witnessing a person revealing and healing himself in such a deep and intimate manner.

Some Self-Revs involve the audience directly, even giving the audience a particular task, highlighting the audience function of participating in the performer's healing. One performer instructed the audience to ask her, 'How are you feeling in your body?,' whenever she entered a particular spot on the stage. She would at that point slow down and respond spontaneously to this question. As her piece included a segment of reliving a traumatic event in her childhood, this here-and-now reconnection to herself and to the audience was not only therapeutically helpful, but also further cemented the audience's sense of traveling through this journey with her. Less commonly, performers have broken the fourth wall by relating directly to a particular person in the audience. Claudia Cuentas Oviedo, in *Canta Corazón* (2010), spoke in Spanish to her actual mother who was seated in the audience, during a latter segment of her piece. While many in the audience could not comprehend the actual words, it was clear that she was speaking tenderly, as she held a scarf wrapped as a swaddled baby representing her own inner child. She was honoring her mother, and at the same time claiming her own responsibility for taking caring of and nurturing her (Claudia's) wounds. Other performances have at first appeared to address particular members in the audience or audience members have come onto to the stage, but moments later it became clear that they were in fact actors, in the role of central players in the performer's life.

While the audience generally feels very involved in the actions on the stage (Sajnani, 2012), there can also be striking ways in which the audience can feel on the outskirts; the performer is seemingly oblivious of the audience and focused just on herself. In actuality, though, the aesthetic of the piece and its capacity to communicate to an audience should never be overlooked or sacrificed. However, the performer may be engaged in some very vulnerable moments within the piece, and using a form that works best for her therapeutically and emotionally. For example, some performers will switch—at a key moment—to speaking in their native language. In a Phase Three or Four scene within a drama therapy session (Emunah, 1994, 2009), using one's native language will at times help the client connect more fully and emotionally to the scene, or be enabled to speak words that stem from an earlier time in her life or a more primal part of her psyche. When this language-switch occurs within a performance, the performer typically becomes underdistanced (Landy, 1986), and her affect in fact heightens the audience's engagement. Usually, these moments are brief but highly poignant. The audience also further grasps at such moments the cultural and language dimensions to the performer's experience. In *Unseen Thread*, Yahuei Chi (2012) slowly unwrapped the cords of a marionette doll which represented herself and the ways she felt externally controlled throughout her life. When she cradled and began gently speaking to the now un-corded doll, it was in her native Mandarin, which released deep-seated emotions in this pivotal healing point in her piece.

At the same that audiences should not be burdened, it is important that the performer consider how much power she allocates to the audience. Although the audience's witnessing becomes interlinked with the healing potential of the piece for the performer, the piece itself should not be overly reliant on the audience. In developing her Self-Rev, one performer—whose piece dealt with the lingering blow of her mother's death when the performer was a 14-year-old girl—considered asking the audience at one point in the piece to state words they thought her mother would say to her now. While this might have been powerful, it was also risky, due to the therapeutic importance of discovering for herself what she needed to hear, and internalizing these words (compounded by the intricacies of adolescent guilt she had been left with at the time of loss). As I was collaborating with her and her director, I suggested that she find and speak her own lines, which she ultimately did, and which led to a theatrically and therapeutically heartrending moment on stage.

Self-Rev and Self-indulgence

Both the term Self-Rev and the description of Self-Rev can evoke valid concerns about self-indulgence. Recent eras have overly emphasized the self, while paying less attention to creating needed change—societally, environmentally, and globally. Performers and directors of Self-Revs should be attentive to the potential pitfall of Self-Revs becoming self-indulgent. In strong Self-Revs, the personal has universal reverberations, and the performer's emotionality strikes resonant chords in that of audience members. Moreover, skillful Self-Revs shed light onto critical social issues. One examines oneself in context. Expanding perspective is key in Self-Rev. There is both a burrowing into deeply personal experience *and* an extending outward toward wider implications.

Autobiographical performance, which runs the same risk of self-indulgence, in fact has had a long history of connecting the personal with the political. The surge of autobiographical performances in the 1970s was tied to consciousness-raising activities related in particular to feminism (Heddon, 2008). A majority of autobiographical performances have been concerned with 'making visible denied or marginalized subjects... aiming to challenge, contest, and problematize dominant representations and assumptions about these subjects' (Heddon, 2008, p. 20). Most therapeutic theatre performances also challenge assumptions and stereotypes, largely by having people in marginalized or stigmatized societal positions put on shows about who they are beneath the ways they are outwardly perceived, as well as by depicting the obstacles they face, their resiliency, their universal yearnings, and the ways in which their concerns are collective human concerns (Emunah & Johnson, 1983; Snow, D'Amico, & Tanguay, 2003). This was certainly true of *Beyond Analysis*, a theatre company I directed for ex-psychiatric patients (Emunah, 1994).

In a theatre review, entitled *The Thin Line*, of one Beyond Analysis production, *Inside Out*, theatre critic Michael Gallantz pointed to a central matter: 'The most provocative question raised by *Inside Out* may be one raised only indirectly: When does real life turn into art? It's a question we might not even think about because the show does have much theatrical skill and ingenuity... But the production gains intensity from the knowledge that the people on stage are for the most part telling their real life stories...' (Gallantz, 1981, p. 28, also in Emunah, 1994, p. 291). *Inside Out* was a therapeutic theatre production which bordered on Self-Rev. (I had not yet initiated the term Self-Rev in the field, and additionally the show had autobiographical and sociodramatic components.) The review addressed the potentially blurry border between life and art, self-indulgence and artistic transcendence.

The intermingling of the personal with larger social spheres that have bearing on the personal result in multidimensional theatre pieces with depth and breadth. The analysis of the intersections between the personal and sociopolitical leads to products that are both moving and enlightening. Self-Revs have investigated the multigenerational transmission of trauma including post-traumatic slave syndrome (Degruy, 2005) and the psychological reverberations of the Holocaust; the ways in which experiences of discrimination, internalized oppression, and self-esteem interface; and the multilayered impact of violence against women. Many Self-Revs have dealt with the complexities of cultural expectations, responsibilities, and ties. One young Indian woman explored her quest for her own identity, in light of cultural expectations as an Indian woman passed onto her by her mother and grandmother; the different masks she wore both in India and currently in the USA; and the conflict between feeling both lovingly tied to her mother and grandmother but also acting in defiance of the cultural norms for women to which they adhered. Another woman explored her deep connection to her Hassidic roots and yet the ways in which it collided with her bisexuality; the navigation between embracing and rejecting her past; the multiple 'bi's in her life; and her desire for acceptance and wholeness. She sang Hassidic melodies to her own lyrics, evoking an ambiance and profundity that music within a Self-Rev often confers.

Self-disclosure is an obvious component of Self-Rev. Performer and director work at ascertaining what is essential to reveal within the piece, without overwhelming either the performer or the audience with unnecessary details. Most importantly, the focus on what to do with the disclosed material (rather than on disclosing more) helps steer the product in an inclusive direction. There is wisdom and universality in seeing how people handle and transform personal struggles.

The emphases in Self-Revs on theatrical quality, and on change and healing, help circumvent self-indulgence. By contrast, self-indulgence is marked by repetition and limiting self-centeredness—which obstruct awareness and artistry. Underlying Self-Rev is an insistence on artistically serving the audience. While the dual focus on both process and product can at times be a tense juggling act, more often aesthetic and therapeutic dimensions and decisions coincide or complement each other (Emunah, 1994). Even in process-oriented drama therapy, attentiveness to aesthetics is relevant (Emunah, 1994; Pendzik, 2013). In Self-Rev performance, theatrical mastery is critical.

Contextualizing one's personal struggles within a cultural and multigenerational context, understanding the perspectives of other players in one's life, delving into psychological complexities, examining the intricacies of our human emotions and our multidimensionality, and creating a work of artistic quality, all steer Self-Revs away from self-indulgence. Ultimately, the most important aspect that leads Self-Revs away from self-indulgence and toward universality and connectedness is the process of grappling with and ultimately transforming inner turmoil, via our generative life force.

Conclusion

In strong Self-Revs, audience members are often in a state of suspense, wondering how the performer could possibly heal or even approach the presented struggles. At a drama therapeutic moment, they begin thinking, 'ah, here is the healing.' But several moments later, new angles, resistances, ramifications are depicted, deconstructed, and grappled with; the audience realizes the superficiality of the first healing moment, and that there will be more layers of healing to come within the piece. The emphasis on psychological depth augments the theatrical power of Self-Revs. And for the performer, theatrical achievement is potently interlaced with personal healing.

My hope is that with an awareness of the power and potentiality of Self-Rev, as well as of its potential caveats, which include self-indulgence, the form will continue to develop and thrive. I have attempted in this chapter to explicate the process of developing a Self-Rev performance, and to articulate the nuances for the performer of being witnessed by an audience, as well as the impact on the audience of beholding such an intimate, if not sacred, theatrical act.

References

Blatner, A. (1988). *Acting-in* (2nd ed.). New York: Springer.

Degruy, J. (2005). *Post-traumatic slave syndrome*. Portland, Oregon: Uptone Press.

Ellis, C. (2007). Telling secrets, revealing lives: Relational ethics in research with intimate others. *Qualitative Inquiry, 13*, 3–29.

Emunah, R. (1994). *Acting for real: Drama therapy process, technique, and performance*. New York/London: Routledge/Taylor and Francis (originally Brunner-Mazel).

Emunah, R. (1995). From adolescent trauma to adolescent drama. In S. Jennings (Ed.), *Dramatherapy with children and adolescents* (pp. 150–168). New York/London: Routledge.

Emunah, R. (2009). The integrative five phase model of drama therapy. In D. Johnson & R. Emunah (Eds.), *Current approaches in drama therapy* (2nd ed., pp. 37–64). Springfield, IL: Charles Thomas.

Emunah, R. (2015). Self-revelatory performance: A form of drama therapy and theatre. *Drama Therapy Review, 1*(1), 71–85.

Emunah, R., & Johnson, D. (1983). The impact of theatrical performance on the self-images of psychiatric patients. *Arts in Psychotherapy, 10*, 233–239.

Emunah, R., Raucher, G., & Ramirez, A. (2014). Self-revelatory performance in mitigating the impact of trauma. In N. Sajnani & D. Johnson (Eds.), *Trauma informed drama therapy* (pp. 93–121). Springfield, IL: Charles Thomas.

Gallantz, M. (1981). *ArtBeat Magazine*, p. 28. (no longer in print).

Heddon, D. (2008). *Autobiography and performance*. New York: Palgrave Macmillan.

Landy, R. (1986). *Drama therapy: Concepts and practices*. Springfield, IL: Charles Thomas.

Pendzik, S. (2013). The 6-key model and the assessment of the aesthetic dimension in dramatherapy. *Dramatherapy, 35*(2), 90–98.

Poulous, C. (2009). *Accidental ethnography*. Walnut Creek, CA: Left Coast Press.

Sajnani, N. (2012). The implicated witness: Towards a relational aesthetic in dramatherapy. *Dramatherapy, 34*(1), 5–20.

Snow, S., D'Amico, M., & Tanguay, D. (2003). Therapeutic theatre and well-being. *Arts in Psychotherapy, 30*(2), 73–82.

SELF-REV PERFORMANCES (AND PERFORMER'S REFLECTIONS)[1]

Chi, Y. (2012). *Unseen Thread*. Director: J. Sopko.

Cuentis, C. (2010). *Canta Corazon*. Director: S. Rubin and G. Hoffman Soto.

Kilman, E. (2009). *This is about Heartbreak*. Director: C. Kammler.

Lemoult, D. (2011). *Mal de Mer*. Director: S. Rubin.

Mazaris, J. (2008). *Little Miss Self*. Director: C. Lewis.

Smith, D. (2012). *Root*. Director: C. Lewis.

Snoddy, M. (2011). *The Buzzing Broken Beat of Life*. Director: S. Trotter.

Toth, J. (2011). *Inner World Lullabies*. Director: C. Lewis.

NOTE

1. All performers referred to by name in this chapter have given their permission.

CHAPTER 4

The Dramaturgy of Autobiographical Therapeutic Performance

Susana Pendzik

For over twenty years I have accompanied *autobiographical therapeutic performances* (ATP) in a variety of contexts, including drama therapy programs, group and individuals in private practice—and have also gone through the process myself. Although each journey is unique, I have observed several patterns that tend to recur, forming the basis of what I call the *dramaturgy of autobiographical therapeutic performance*. This chapter reflects on some of the main aspects involved in this dramaturgy, in terms of both the process, and also of the pieces created under its guidance and inspiration.

THERAPEUTIC DRAMATURGY

In western theatre, dramaturgy has been traditionally associated with playwriting. In its classical sense, it deals with the constitutive elements of play construction and is defined as 'the art of composition of plays' (Pavis, 1998, p. 124). However, the term was subsequently broadened to incor-

S. Pendzik, PhD, MA, RDT (✉)
Tel Hai Academic College, Upper Galilee, Israel

Hebrew University of Jerusalem, Jerusalem, Israel

Swiss Institute of Dramatherapy, St Gallen, Switzerland
e-mail: pend@netvision.net.il

© The Author(s) 2016
S. Pendzik et al. (eds.), *The Self in Performance*,
DOI 10.1057/978-1-137-53593-1_4

55

porate the play's staging as a performance; and expanded (inspired by the ideas of Brecht) to include not only the formal but also the ideological structures of playwriting, staging, and production (Lehmann, 2006). This paved the way for a discussion of dramaturgy that embraces its pedagogical, interpretative, political, and power-related implications (Amkpa, 2006; Bogad, 2006).

The way I use the concept of dramaturgy is attuned to Eugenio Barba's (2010) formulations. In his view, far from being mainly concerned with narrative composition, dramaturgy involves an operation that is 'inherent in the weaving and growth of a performance and its different components' (p. 8). Barba looks at performance as a living organism, seeing not only its parts, but also the layers they create, their complex organization, and the mutual relationships established. He concludes that dramaturgy is like 'anatomy' (2010, p. 9), and identifies three different levels in it: the *organic dramaturgy*—the elementary level of physical embodiment; the *narrative*—the meaning-producing intertwining of events; and the *evocative* level—the one that resonates in the spectators. In this chapter, I deal mainly with the first two levels. (I briefly refer to the third in Pendzik, 2013a.)

Although Barba (2010) expresses the perspective of a theatre director with no therapeutic aims, some of his ideas may be applicable in the context of ATP. Particularly illuminating are his views on the creative process and the created product as configurations and patterns that are reproduced at all levels. Product and process are two strands of the same embroidery and the dramaturgy of the first is intrinsically and organically connected to that of the latter.

Working on a performance invariably presents performers with a series of challenges, ranging from technical and structural to aesthetic and conceptual. These become exacerbated when the performance is based on personal material. Yet lurking around these challenges is where old and unhelpful patterns of dealing with life can be found, confronted, and changed. I have observed that some of these challenges take particular forms; and although there are many ways of handling them, what I call *therapeutic dramaturgy* offers insightful and transformative possibilities, which involve taking balanced risks, opening up emotionally, expanding role repertoire, allowing complexity and paradox to be expressed, and envisioning change. Sometimes these processes unfold naturally as a by-product of the artistic work—akin to Winnicott's (2005) notion of healthy play being itself the therapy. However, the pull towards regressive patterns often takes over the process; and that's when non-therapeutic and therapeutic dramaturgies depart: An ATP dramaturgy implies going beyond the staging of personal narratives, involving a process of self-exploration and discovery that aims at transformation and change.

For logistic reasons I separate the configurations encountered in ATP dramaturgy into those that are more concerned with the process and those appearing in the play itself; I do this while keeping in mind that, as a living organism, the patterns of form/content/process/product will repeat themselves and resonate in different levels.

MILESTONES IN THE DRAMATURGY OF ATP

Leaps into the Unknown: Openings vs. A Priori Structures

According to Susanne Langer (1953), the function of art is to acquaint the beholder with something s/he 'has not known before' (p. 19). ATP is both an artistic and a psychotherapeutic journey. Individuals embarking on it may have ideas, desires, or assumptions as to where the road may lead them—just as we anticipate, when setting out on a voyage, the adventures awaiting us. Some regard this journey as an opportunity to confront aspects of their life that have been waiting for a chance to emerge; others fantasize about taking another opportunity to elaborate old issues that still feel unresolved; people may even play some scenes in their minds that they would like to see staged. These a priori ideas may be engaging; yet they also constitute one the first dangers encountered in the journey, for often these initial wishes are embedded with old values or ruled by the conventions and aesthetics of what narrative therapy calls the *dominant story* (White & Epston, 1990). If there is self-discovery in this process, entering it means precisely *not knowing too much.*

Many scholars refer to the entrance into the unknown as an essential step of the creative/therapeutic process. Joseph Campbell (2004) emphasizes that the adventures of the hero often begin in a way that the 'individual is drawn into a relationship with forces that are not rightly understood' (p. 46). Linda Schierse-Leonard (2009) speaks about the first stage in a creative project as a 'time of surrender... to take a leap into the unknown' (p. 7). Victor Turner (1982) conceives the liminal phase, as a place of 'ambiguity, a sort of social limbo' (p. 24) that may be experienced as disorienting, but also as potentially transformative, while Erika Fischer-Lichte (2002) links the liminal in both theatre and transition ritual 'with the creation, self-fashioning and transformation of identity' (p. 4). Similar ideas impregnate the work of Jerzy Grotowski (1968), for whom the state of mind required for the creation of the performer's *total act* is a 'passive readiness... a state in which one "does not want to do that" but rather "resigns from not doing it"' (p. 17). In a similar vein, Barba (2000) utilizes a *technique of disorientation* that 'consists in giving space to a multiplicity of trends, narratives and directions without bending them, right from the start, beneath the yoke of our choices and intentions' (p. 60); and Tami Spry (2011) teaches her autoethnography students to focus on *practiced vulnerability*, 'a methodology for moving out of one's comfort zone of familiarity, a strategic surrendering into a space of risk, of uncomfortability, of uncertainty that one experiences when critically reflecting upon and then embodying one's own experience' (p. 167).

The dramaturgy of ATP often brings people to experience this kind of disorienting, indeterminate state. Even if they started by working on an a priori idea or re-telling a story they know about themselves, individuals may suddenly find there is another story unfolding. Usually, this is not a completely foreign one, but one that they recognize has been waiting to come out, eliciting feelings of serendipity, insight or revelation—akin to what Johnson (Chap. 5) calls *surprise*. For many people, the encounter with unseen aspects of themselves constitutes a significant twist in their personal process, bringing about a sense of release. For example, a woman who had assumed she would be doing yet another cycle of work around a central traumatic event in her life, realized that she was not bound to deal with this issue repeatedly, and that as far as she was concerned, the truly therapeutic intervention was to move on to other aspects of her life. This insight released her from a narrow perception of herself and gave her the freedom to reframe her identity beyond her trauma.

There is ample space for therapeutic work in this stage; for the invitation to run into autobiographical aspects that are not in our 'conscious list' promotes self-discovery and challenges discourses that we have repeated to ourselves—thus validating marginal ones. At the same time, having one's main storyline shattered can be disorienting or upsetting for individuals who are too concerned with the end product or are invested in making a point. This is solid therapeutic material to work with, and—consonant with Emunah's (2015) *working through* concept—illustrates that therapeutic dramaturgy is not equal with staging one's life experiences. Because ATP is a therapeutic journey, any feelings elicited by it are accounted for and incorporated into the process.

Closely resembling Barba's (2000) technique of disorientation or Spry's (2011) practiced vulnerability, I use an approach that I call *openings* in order to facilitate the loosening of constructs that is necessary to initiate any creative cycle (Kelly, 1991). Openings are performed over five to seven sessions in which several aspects of the person's life are tackled from a variety of angles, using different techniques, in an attempt to keep the beginning of the process as an expansive and fluid exploration (Pendzik, 2013a). For instance, one session may focus on ancestry, using family trees or folk songs as prompts, while the next may deal with current life conflicts and be based on embodied images and movement techniques. Sessions are viewed as single units—an approach that allows for the exploration of multiple narratives, rather than fixing the work on a single topic from the start. I encourage participants to let go of their a priori ideas, reassuring them that these will reappear if they really are the ones that ought to go on stage.

By the time this phase comes to an end, several aspects emerge as leading issues, themes or motifs that need to be addressed, which had not necessarily been anticipated. Discovering untapped, less explored facets of the self may carry the power of a revelation: Some people describe this as emotionally uplifting—like a paradigm shift experienced on a personal level. As in the creativity cycle model, this stage is often marked by the outpouring of artistic ideas, material, and feelings that also lead to further insights (Gordon, 1995). This creative abundance may last longer for some people than for others, but surfing on this wave is only good for a certain time in ATP—as its presentational format requires the material to be moulded into art forms that will be publicly shared. Thus, the enlightening experience initiated by the openings may turn eventually into the *now what* phase, as the process leads participants to search for the appropriate artistic forms that could give expression to the recently discovered material.

Struggles with Form and Content

The dialogue between form and content is always dialectical: Discovering the issue that needs to be dealt with both affects and is affected by the form in which it is presented. Respectively, a meaningful theme can be found through the mediation of an aesthetic form, or both content and form may find each other in a majestic, synchronous stroke. Be it through a cogent stage metaphor, an accurate genre, or a compelling prop, a charged therapeutic moment occurs when a meaningful issue encounters a suitable aesthetic shape that channels it.

As an example, a woman began the process with the idea of doing a personal adaptation of *Hansel and Gretel*; she felt attracted to the themes of getting lost in the forest, the power relations between the witch and the children, and the forbidden and dangerous passion of eating too many sweets. Although she entered the process *with* the story, this wasn't an a priori idea, as the tale allowed ample space for the exploration of personal meaning within its context. Rather than coming from a conscious list, the knowledge that this particular tale could be a container for childhood experiences of emotional abandonment and social oppression was floating in the back of her mind. She had initially conceived staging the piece by using dolls for the characters (as in a puppet show), and telling the story by moving in and out of the role of narrator. However, as the work advanced, this format proved limiting and barren. In addition, we discovered that the Witch's character was not sufficiently developed and tended to be projected outside of the self. I suggested leaving the puppet plan aside and doing embodied work around the Witch, reassuring her that the previous format could always be reinstated. This was a major therapeutic turning point: Engagement with the Witch overturned the puppet show, challenging as well the author/performer's main identification with the victimization of the children. The character of the Witch voiced issues connected to gender, physical appearance, food intake, and professional achievements. The performance became an embodied show that included the preparation of papier-mâché on stage, using newspapers that symbolized at once the forest of homelessness, women's domestic duties, social pressure and criticism, food, and creativity.

The process of finding the story had been meaningful for this woman; however, the main therapeutic effect was achieved not so much from the story as from struggling with the form in which it needed to be told. Discovering the story could only take her a certain length in her journey. The creative process is always bound to reach a point of impasse where new therapeutic challenges are found.

While developing *Developmental Transformations* (DvT), David Read Johnson (1991) noted the therapeutic importance of the *impasse* in improvisation and pointed at ways in which drama therapists may work with it. In DvT an impasse denotes the quality of being stuck, and is experienced as a disruption in the flow of action that results in confusion, repetition, etc., usually bringing the scene to a dead end. Broadly used, an impasse happens 'any time in treatment when clients struggle to move to another level of development and/or are at the brink of this transition' (Porter, 2003, p. 101).

In ATP dramatic impasses are encountered at every step of the journey; they are experienced each time the person faces a creative block, whenever material is handled using rigid structures or exhausted art forms, when people attach themselves to a particular narrative ('trying to make a point,' 'telling it as it was'), or repeat its content as if in a loop (Pendzik, 2013b). One very common impasse presents itself around 'technical matters'. Although apparently relating to concrete levels of production, technical issues are not devoid of emotional resonance, as they incarnate the materialization of mental structures and other aspects of the individual's inner world. As Pavis (1998) claims, 'meaning in theatre is always a technical issue that has to do with materials, forms and structures' (p. 125), and Peter Brook (1981) concludes even more simply: 'the aesthetics are practical' (p. 98).

To illustrate, at the beginning of the process a middle-aged man had a technical question: 'Would there be a piano for his performance?' When informed that unfortunately a piano could not be brought to the stage, he was unwilling to consider any alternatives. Upset, he insisted on moving the whole production somewhere else (a rather complicated task), claiming he was not going to perform unless there was a real piano on stage. At first glance, his request can be seen as a legitimate artistic or technical one; however, his reaction was so disproportionate that it cried out for clarification. Getting in touch with his feelings revealed the story of the intense pressure that had been exerted on him by his parents to take piano lessons during his childhood. Although he had stopped playing a long time ago, he could not conceive of an autobiographical piece that would not feature a piano on stage. Perhaps in non-therapeutic forms of autobiographical theatre, this issue might have been dealt with by either moving the production or finding a way to bring a piano on stage. However, as in this example, most technical issues encompass an emotional dimension; and in ATP, addressing this aspect is an integral part of the dramaturgy.

Therapeusis of the End: Deus ex Machina *vs. Envisioning an* Horizon

One recurrent challenge (often an impasse) in the dramaturgy of ATP is the difficulty people experience in finding a suitable ending for their piece.

While presenting emotionally charged, personal material in an aesthetic manner brings about a sense of fulfillment and insight, these therapeutic accomplishments are threatened if a meaningful denouement cannot be articulated. Moreover, working against the deadline of a performance exacerbates the feelings of anxiety and frustration that this struggle produces. Elsewhere I have compared ATP to giving birth (Pendzik, 2013a): As the performance approaches, the tension mounts, climaxing in a sense of urgency, of things needing to fall into place on time—or else catastrophe will befall.

Although there are innumerable ways of what Emunah (2015) calls *grappling with* this challenge, in the emotional turmoil of trying to find a good—or even a conceivable—resolution to the piece, people get caught in old patterns of solving things in real life. Paradigmatic of this are endings that resort to *Deus ex Machina* configurations in which an extraordinary or 'unanticipated intervener' (Cuddon, 1991, p. 237) appears and resolves the situation. Not infrequently these are the presenter's life partners, children, etc., so that their wish to be saved is projected upon significant others. In a typical example, traumatic experiences or personal crises are miraculously resolved through the intervention of a character that has no credible basis (plot-wise) or whose entrance is not as well elaborated, dramatically speaking, as the trauma itself. Endings that take the form of a magical way out, in which events are not integral to the plot, are indicative of unresolved issues and call for further therapeutic work. Even Aristotle (1902) criticized the use of this device, claiming that the 'unravelling of the plot… must arise out of the plot itself' and that '*Deus ex Machina* should be employed only for events… which lie beyond the human knowledge' (pp. 55–6).

Additional old patterns include leaving the piece unresolved (the protagonist is bleeding on stage when the curtain falls), repeating the cycle (the scene restarts as the lights go off, implying another merry-go-round), or finishing it abruptly (a sudden blackout in the middle of a distressing situation). Whether compulsive, obsessive or suicidal, there is a lot of acting out in these attempted endings—akin to what drama therapy terms *underdistance,* defined as an 'overabundance of emotionality', or *overdistance,* 'a lack of emotional expression' (Landy, 2008, p. 101). Although these endings sometimes echo the aesthetics of postdramatic theatre (Lehmann, 2006), as we are speaking of a process that is not meant to move or shock the audience, but mainly to achieve therapeusis, the question is what aesthetics should the author/performer pursue? Moreover, the performance is based not only on autobiographical material, but also becomes autobiographical—in the sense that it constitutes an actual experience that will be inscribed in our body/mind/soul; it will be thoroughly rehearsed (including memorizing gestures and words), and publicly validated by the witnessing presence of an audience. Clearly, if a therapeutic accomplishment is to be gained in this process, it is not through the repetition of old patterns (which may be re-traumatizing even if they are aesthetically thought-provoking), but in the opportunity for repair that it offers (Emunah, 2015). As Moreno (1972) claims regarding the re-enactment of life scenes in psychodrama, the emphasis should not be placed on imitation of life 'but upon the opportunity of recapitulation of unresolved problems' that it permits (p. 15). Here is an example:

Basing the piece on her diary as a teenager, one woman included a fragment that referred to a sexual assault perpetrated on her by a charming man who had also been her boss. She had never before defined this experience as sexual assault, and it was only through the ATP group work that she began to confront, reframe, and process the event. She resolutely decided to stand alone on stage, presenting the piece as a monologue; her suggested ending was that the 'lights go off abruptly as the man is about to assault her.' The feedback she got from group members, my co-facilitator, and myself, was that this shocking conclusion would leave everyone in a state of perplexity and distress. Yet she replied that she purposely 'wanted the audience to experience exactly' what she felt. Being an actress, she also thought that this ending would be very suitable in a theatrical setting. I told her that the focus in ATP is less on what the audience feels than on what she needs to process about this experience, and invited her to consider other ending options. After many trials that did not work for her, almost a day before the performance she came up with a brilliant stage image: The lights go off, and after a few moments they go on again, showing her running on the spot, facing the audience, while a song by a famous female singer is being played that speaks about freedom, hope, and empowerment for women. One by one, group members join her, running with her as they look at each other supportively, creating a reassuring connection, until the stage is filled with a powerful group of running women. This ending brought the piece to a different level of integration, achieving not only a therapeutic aim for the protagonist, but also generating a collective resonance that included the group and the audience—as personal and public became united.

In a follow-up interview one year later, the protagonist recognized the remarkable impact of this intervention, and as I turned to her again to write this chapter, she wrote about that ending:

> ... a resonant effect goes with me over the past few years, that turned something closed and dark into something open, full of sharing, and power; and because of that good closing scene in my ATP... I feel there is feminine strength within me, as the power of women friends running together accompanies me—and I can hold the complexity of it (personal communication).

In ATP, the translation of personal experiences into stage language is not only a means to express pain or beauty, or to challenge the audience. Its main purpose is to allow the experiences to be processed, to undergo transformation, to evolve. Therefore, ATP denouements need to have what I call a *therapeutic horizon*—something that gives the situation presented 'a range of perception, a scope, a view, or even a hint of what becomes' (Pendzik, 2013a, p. 20). Since not every situation can have—nor would we wish it to have—a happy ending, we need not confuse the notion of therapeutic horizon with the imperative of finding a merry solution. A piece with therapeutic horizon tends to bring forth a sense of hopefulness that does not derive from a quick fix or a clichéd ending; sometimes the hopeful hint is implied in the acceptance of a situation that is irrevocable or beyond recall. As in the above mentioned piece, a therapeutic horizon often elicits profound resonances (Pendzik, 2008) in the author/performer as well as in the audience. Thus, although the invitation to have a therapeutic horizon may have aesthetic implications, its real purpose is to highlight the fact that the presentation itself becomes a significant autobiographical experience, which leaves enduring therapeutic traces in the life of the performer.

Patterns in the Dramaturgy of the Plot

Among the numerous possibilities of weaving ATP plots, I have identified several configurations that tend to recur in what Barba (2010) calls the narrative level of dramaturgy. Two of these constellations are the *oppression/liberation paradigm* and the *search archetype*—or journey. These general categorizations may appear in a variety of combinations as well.

The oppression/liberation paradigm comprises a dramaturgical arrangement that often begins in the oppressive pole: The person is exploited, abused, neglected, bullied or tyrannized either by significant others (parents, siblings, peers) or by inner aspects of themselves (inner critic, cynical self). In one example, an overpowering mother is represented by two characters that interfere with the protagonist's lines, constantly correcting her, speaking in her name, and intruding in every attempt she makes to tell a story. Gradually, the protagonist becomes a puppet on strings, and the two mothers—standing on high platforms—manipulate her, as she tries to tell a tale about a puppet that wanted to go places but stayed in one spot. A liberating breakthrough comes as the puppet in the tale discovers that she has a heart, from which grows a pair of flying wings. This realization has an immediate impact, both upon the mothers who freeze in terror, and upon the puppet, who eventually removes the strings and walks away as a human being, sending the mothers a farewell kiss from a distance.

The acts of liberation take many forms: growing up, leaving, getting a voice, disentangling oneself from knots, breaking away from prisons, etc. Many use stage metaphors involving the body—in resonance with Spry's (2011) assertions about the complex role of the body in autoethnographic performance: body-as-evidence and body-of-evidence. For example, in an ATP that used an adaptation of *Cinderella*, the sisters are presented as a pair of Barbie dolls who exploit and humiliate the protagonist, while dancing mechanically to the tune of *Barbie Girl* and speaking in distorted voices. As the protagonist is left on stage to clean and cook, a fairy comes in and tries to tell her how beautiful and special she is, but Cinderella ignores her, not even looking at her face. Two birds appear, dancing the Beatles' *Blackbird* song, and Cinderella—first hesitantly and then wholeheartedly—joins them, gradually developing the sweeping movements into a free dance involving the whole body. Through the dance she liberates herself from the roles of Barbie and Cinderella, until she finally is able to embody the Prince that chooses her as a bride.

The search or journey constellation is less of an arc, tending rather to be organized as a spiral or in curves—like epic theatre. In the following example, the piece begins with a man listening to a recording of himself reciting from the Bible as he prepares for his Bar Mitzvah. In an imaginary dialogue with his father, he fancies asking him about his childhood in Morocco; and putting on his father's jacket he delivers a monologue (in Arabic) that might have been voiced by his father. The next scene opens with three adolescents idling away and 'inventing cool trends,' pretending to play the guitar. The protagonist erupts on stage as an adolescent, wearing 'the wrong clothes,' as a dramatic song by a well-known singer identified with Oriental (non-European) Jews is played. The three idlers make derogatory comments about him; but as the scene unfolds, the protagonist becomes their leader, fashioning the new trends as they copy everything he does. The third scene shows a visit to the protagonist's grandmother, who feeds him with her special (ethnic) food, while telling him stories about the ancestors. As she narrates these folk tales, her body recreates daily tasks such as cooking, washing clothes, or praying, as a dance. The protagonist imitates her movements as they dance together to North African music; after a while, Grandma kisses him goodbye and exits the stage for good (passes away), leaving him alone and confused. In the fourth scene a young woman enters the stage, dancing to a different music; a duet develops between them in which he tries to chase her and she disappears or flees every time he is about to catch her. Finally, he discovers a way of dancing with her that is not power-driven and they dance together until she exits. Alone on stage, he keeps on dancing in a free form, on his own, joyfully.

In this piece we recognize many elements of epic theatre aesthetics and dramaturgy (Brecht, 1981): Each scene stands on its own, the development is in curves, there are jumps between scenes; the narrative explores an issue more than telling a particular story; and, of course, there is an invitation to look at the piece from a critical and political context. Although there might be a liberating element in it, what moves the piece is the search: searching for father, for roots, for identity.

In some cases, the two configurations—oppression/liberation and search—combine. To illustrate, a woman enacts herself as a little girl whose parents play games with each other (instead of playing with her). This situation repeats itself as a series of entrances and exits of her parents: Father goes in and out of the stage riding on a scooter (each time with a different woman); mother is too busy, always running. At a climatic point the protagonist stops the cycle, shouting: 'I don't understand the games that adults play...!'—followed by a tenebrous monologue with suicidal undertones. In the following scene she is at the Gates of Heaven, where the Vice-God is mending a broken scooter at the top of a ladder. Recognizing her father's scooter, she requests from the Vice-God to let her in. He replies that it's not her time yet, and a dialogue unfolds between them. In the end, she asks him to allow her to lay her head on his shoulder. He agrees and she stays there, resting for some moments; then slowly begins to walk down the ladder, as the lights go dim.

The first part of this piece exemplifies the oppression/liberation para-digm: A sense of crescendo builds up in the recurring and increasingly quicker entrances of the parents, and the protagonist explodes in a sui-cidal monologue. The scene at the Gates of Heaven, on the other hand, belongs to the aesthetics of the search: It stands as a unit, has a reflective quality, is more poetic than dramatic, and lacks the cathartic edge that characterizes the oppression liberation/paradigm.

These two archetypal configurations are very common in ATP—although I do not imply they are the only ones. Plots may be arranged in other patterns, such as *life cycles*, in which the piece is woven as a sequence of seasons or life phases (Galila Oren, personal communication), *past and present parallels*, where scenes of 'then and now' are analogized and played against each other (Chen Alon, personal communication); or in the form of *memorials* or other ritual structures.

Closure

The oppression/liberation and the search configurations seem to play a role in all three levels of dramaturgy mentioned by Barba (2010): the organic or dynamic level (the body, rhythms, movement, senses); the nar-rative (which I detailed in the last section); and the evocative ('the faculty of the performance to produce an intimate resonance within the spectator' (p. 10)). They reflect the two dramaturgic veins that run deep in western theatre, the epic and the cathartic, epitomized in the twentieth century by the works of Brecht and Artaud, respectively. They furthermore con-stitute central aspects of the process of rehearsal and performance: open-ings, for example, seem more attuned to the search archetype, whereas the impasse and the horizon are more inclined toward the oppression/ liberation paradigm.

This chapter has focused on the dramaturgy of the author/performer. Barba (2010) proposes that besides the dramaturgy of the actor, there are also those of the director and the spectators. This is certainly true of ATP, where the therapist/director (typically a drama therapist) is inti-mately engaged in accompanying a process of which s/he is not an equal co-creator. The therapist/director's dramaturgy is about midwifery in all its complexity; it is concerned with channeling a living organism into life (Pendzik, 2013a). The spectators' dramaturgy is connected to the reso-nant layer that the personal and the collective realms activate in each other. On the one hand, their dramaturgy is about recreating the experience of *communitas* (Turner, 1982) that ATP can offer; on the other, as Jacques Rancière (2009) suggests, it is about embodying an emancipated community of individuals, each of whom allows the performance to resonate with their own stories.

REFERENCES

Amkpa, A. (2006). Re-envisioning theatre, activism, and citizenship in neocolonial contexts. In J. Cohen Cruz & M. Schutzman (Eds.), *A Boal companion: Dialogues on theatre and cultural politics* (pp. 161–172). London: Routledge.
Aristotle. (1902). *Poetics* (Transl. S. H. Butcher, 3rd ed.). London: Macmillan.
Barba, E. (2000). The deep order called turbulence: The three faces of dramaturgy. *The Drama Review, 44*(4), 56–66.
Barba, E. (2010). *On directing and dramaturgy.* London: Routledge.
Bogad, L. M. (2006). Tactical carnival: Social movements, demonstrations and dialogical performance. In J. Cohen Cruz & M. Schutzman (Eds.), *A Boal companion: Dialogues on theatre and cultural politics* (pp. 46–58). London: Routledge.
Brecht, B. (1981). The modern theatre is the epic theatre. In J. Willet (Ed. and Trans.), *Brecht on theatre* (pp. 33–43). London: Methuen.
Brook, P. (1981). *The empty space.* New York: Atheneum.
Campbell, J. (2004). *The hero with a thousand faces.* Princeton: Princeton University Press.
Cuddon, J. A. (1991). *Dictionary of literary terms and literary theory.* London: Penguin.
Emunah, R. (2015). Self-revelatory performance: A form of drama therapy and theatre. *Drama Therapy Review, 1*(1), 71–85.
Fischer-Lichte, E. (2002). *History of European drama and theatre.* London and New York: Routledge.
Gordon, R. (1995). *Bridges: Psychic structures, functions, and processes.* New Brunswick, NJ: Transaction Publishers.
Grotowski, J. (1968). *Towards a poor theatre.* New York: Simon & Schuster.
Johnson, D. R. (1991). The theory and technique of transformations in drama therapy. *Arts in Psychotherapy, 18*, 285–300.
Kelly, G. A. (1991). *The psychology of personal constructs.* London: Routledge.
Landy, R. (2008). *The couch and the stage.* Lanham, MD: Jason Aronson.
Langer, S. (1953). *Feeling and form.* New York: Charles Scribner's Sons.
Lehmann, H. T. (2006). *Postdramatic theatre.* London: Routledge.
Moreno, J. L. (1972). *Psychodrama* (Vol. 1, 3rd ed.). New York: Beacon Press.
Pavis, P. (1998). *Dictionary of the theatre: Terms, concepts, and analysis.* Toronto: University of Toronto Press.

Pendzik, S. (2008). Dramatic resonances: A technique of intervention in drama therapy, supervision, and training. *Arts in Psychotherapy, 35*, 217–223.

Pendzik, S. (2013a). The poiesis and praxis of autobiographical therapeutic theatre. Keynote speech, *13th Summer Academy of the German Association of Theatre-Therapy* (DGFT), Remscheid, Germany. https://www.researchgate.net/publication/280530475_

Pendzik, S. (2013b). The 6-Key model and the assessment of the aesthetic dimension in dramatherapy. *Dramatherapy, 35*(2), 90–98. http://dx.doi.org/10.1080/02630672.2013.822524

Porter, L. (2003). Death in transformation: The importance of impasse in drama therapy. *Arts in Psychotherapy, 30*, 101–107.

Rancière, J. (2009). *The emancipated spectator.* London/New York: Verso.

Schierse-Leonard, L. (2009). *The call to create.* New Orleans, LA: Spring Journal Books.

Spry, T. (2011). *Body, paper, stage: Writing and performing autoethnography.* Walnut Creek, CA: Left Coast Press.

Turner, V. (1982). *From ritual to theatre: The human seriousness of play.* New York: PAJ.

White, M., & Epston, D. (1990). *Narrative means to therapeutic ends.* New York & London: W.W. Norton & Company.

Winnicott, D. W. (2005). *Playing and reality.* New York: Routledge.

CHAPTER 5

Surprise and Otherness in Self-revelatory Performance

David Read Johnson

If the essential distinguishing feature of *self-revelatory performance* (Self-Rev) as defined by Renée Emunah (2015) is that the actor is *working through* current issues both during the rehearsal and performance phases, instead of merely presenting autobiographical material, then it is incumbent that a firm understanding of the concept of working through is achieved. Though it is assumed that a certain degree of working through takes place during the preparatory phases and rehearsals, as a collaborative process between actor and director, Emunah posits that working through also takes place during the performance; otherwise the performance would technically be an autobiographical performance about a previously completed therapeutic process. The actor's real emotional presence and vulnerability are crucial components in a Self-Rev performance that distinguish it from standard theatre (Emunah, 2015).

Autobiographical (AP) and *autoethnographic* (AEP) performances consist respectively of either the personal or sociocultural background of the actor, and may or may not be therapeutic. Nontherapeutic forms of per-

D.R. Johnson, PhD, RDT-BCT (✉)
Post-Traumatic Stress Center, New Haven, CT, USA

Department of Psychiatry, Yale University School of Medicine, New Haven, CT, USA
e-mail: davidreadjohnson@gmail.com

© The Author(s) 2016
S. Pendzik et al. (eds.), *The Self in Performance*,
DOI 10.1057/978-1-137-53593-1_5

formance are explicitly intended to *impact the audience*, either through education or entertainment. Self-Rev performance, on the other hand, is explicitly therapeutic in intent, and therefore the director serves to some degree in the role of a therapist, and many audience members have a personal relationship with the actor. Self-Rev intends to *impact the actor as well as the audience*. Actor, director, and audience therefore straddle dual roles based on the performance and therapeutic elements of Self-Rev.

Powerful AP and AEP performances can be intense, personal, emotive, and inspirational, but for the audience. Effective Self-Rev performances must also have this impact on the actor. Self-Rev performances reach for a sense of immediacy and presence reminiscent of Artaud's famous image of actors 'being like victims burnt at the stake, signaling through the flames' (Artaud, 1958, p. 13). This is no small task, since if the Self-Rev performance is moving and inspirational mostly for the actor rather than for the audience, this can result in a self-indulgent and maudlin performance.

Therefore in a Self-Rev, the actor must be subject to the process of discovery. Since most Self-Revs are scrupulously rehearsed and ultimately scripted, where is the room for unexpected developments to occur? How do we conceive of a process of discovery that occurs in the moment of a rehearsed performance? How do we surprise ourselves? There must be an interesting and exquisite relationship between the actor and the script such that openings are allowed for new awareness and unexpected events to emerge. If so, what is that exquisite arrangement and is it any different from the essentials of good acting, in which the actor breathes life into an inert script?

It is hardly sufficient to claim that working through occurs during the performance solely on the basis of self-reports of actors. For Self-Rev to become a recognized and solid therapeutic form, the process of working through must be well understood and theoretically grounded. That is the purpose of this chapter.

Arthur Koestler (1964) famously noted that the fact that we cannot tickle ourselves—and yet we are tickled—is proof of the existence of other people. Tickling evokes feelings of alarm and the desire to get away, and simultaneously feelings of delight and uncontrollable laughter. Koestler goes further in observing that a real tickle is always followed by a pretend tickle, which magically arouses the same and equally intense reaction. He proposes that this response to the pretend tickle may be our first experience of theatre. Indeed, our authentic response to the pretend tickle may be a perfect example of 'living truthfully under imaginary circumstances'

(Meisner & Longwell, 1987), of bringing the *as if* to life. This moment is not only theatrical, it is magical, for something (our reaction) arises out of nothing (mere pretense). It is also comic, even clownish, as we shout 'stop it!' to the other's mere moving their fingers near our body. Tickling is the presence of the Other in its full freedom: we recoil from that which touches us wherever it desires.

If we cannot tickle ourselves, that is, be Other to ourselves, then must we rely on an Other in any process of discovery? Perhaps there are internal sources of Otherness as well? Can we not spontaneously have an 'Aha!' moment? Can we not arrive at new insights by ourselves through processes of deep study and meditation? And, if so, from where do these new insights and ideas come? If healing, or working through, is to occur in Self-Rev, something new must arise in the actor/client; it cannot be known already. It is my contention that the creation of presence, of aliveness, of surprise in the process of working through is reliant on accessing one or more sources of Otherness. Let us now examine the possible sources, both internal and external, of Otherness within the Self-Rev process.

SOURCES OF OTHERNESS IN THE SELF-REV PROCESS

First there is our *individual unconscious and subconscious*. The unconscious is that which is Other to our persona, which includes both personal memories and thoughts and feelings that have been forgotten or suppressed, as well as fantasies, desires, and images that arise in the moment but which are not allowed to enter full consciousness. Presumably in the preparatory phase of a Self-Rev, through personal reflection and embodied and dramatic exploration, by oneself and with the director, unconscious and subconscious aspects of self may rise into awareness, which contribute to the healing process. Nevertheless, it seems more complex to understand how the discovery and processing of unconscious material takes place spontaneously during a performance, in the heat of the moment. Any significant new image or awareness with accompanying cognitive processing, if expressed during the performance, will presumably result in significant departure from the established script, as in cases where periods of improvisation are built into the performance. Otherwise, this source of Otherness will most likely exert its influence during the preparatory phase.

Second, there is the *interaction with the director*. Through discussion, witnessing, and direct feedback, the director provides the actor with new perspectives of which they may not have been aware. The actor may feel surprised, confronted, affirmed, or confused by the feedback of the director, allowing a deeper investigation into the central issues.

A third source of Otherness for some Self-Rev performances arises from the use of *stories, myths, fables, or texts* of other authors to provide metaphoric or symbolic frame to the actor's personal work. The positive effect of these stories is often attributed to their innate powers. However, the insights that arise from these stories may be due to the mere fact of their Otherness, which evokes new perspectives on the actor's personal story.

A fourth source of Otherness is the *effect of the stagecraft* itself: props, makeup, costume, lighting, stage manager, timing, blocking. Though largely impersonal, these artistic elements carry their own rules and limitations, which can provide assistance or resistance to the actor's dramatic intentions, forcing in some cases new discoveries and new paths of expression. Being forced by these external circumstances to do something differently, the actor experiences a new approach to an issue. For example, in one of my own Self-Revs, a prop was to be broken, but when I smashed it on the table during rehearsal, it shattered all over the stage in a way that would make it hard to continue to perform. Therefore, I was forced to smash it slowly, more stylistically, which led immediately to a host of new associations to my father's mistreatment of me, which were then incorporated into the action. In another example, an actress was supposed to use the prop of a revolver at a critical moment of the performance; however, she had forgotten to place it under the tablecloth. The moment arrived, she slipped her hand under the tablecloth and discovered it was not there, immediately realized she had forgotten it, looked out at the audience, paused, and then whispered, 'bang,' tearfully and spontaneously introduced new material, and then continued with her rehearsed lines and actions. Because art is desire made manifest, the materials exert their own unique influences on the final artistic product, whether in visual arts, music, dance, or drama. The relationship between the script and in the *mise en scène* is always dynamic, and often results in surprising twists during performances.

Finally, the *audience* is a source of Otherness for the actor. Because so often in Self-Rev, the audience consists of friends, family, and colleagues, and is performed in small stage spaces where the audience's reactions are easily seen, the actor will be impacted in the moment by these responses, which may provide an impetus for altering the performance as it is occurring, and certainly create new states of feeling within the actor. Since the audience will often include people who also have a stake in what the actor is going through, beyond being audience to a performance, the actor may alter the performance in the moment as they notice these friends and family members' reactions. Other audience members may also in the moment shift their attention to these audience members who are the intimates of the actor, and for a moment members of the audience will in fact become performers. Audiences within audiences may emerge and disappear throughout the performance, leading to a heightened sense of immediacy and presence among all participants.

Though these may be the main five sources of Otherness available to the actor in a Self-Rev process, they will probably exert a greater effect during the rehearsal process, and only briefly during the performance itself. We still do not have a good description of what such a moment of discovery looks like during a performance. Is it possible that what we are looking for is not some kind of new behavior on the part of the actor, but an alteration in the relationship between the actor and the audience; an attitude, perhaps, that the audience recognizes as departing from the expected performance? To achieve such a description of the moment of working through, we need a theory of surprise.

A Theory of Surprise

Though the above sources of Otherness are essential in any Self-Rev process, they skirt what may be the most important component of Self-Rev, which Emunah and others seem to be hinting at: the enactment of surprise. To allow elements from an Other source into a performance, one must be open to them. They are not Other if one is in control of them. These elements therefore must surprise us to some degree. They must be experienced, to some degree, as the previously unknown. How does the Self-Rev actor remain open to these experiences during a performance? To this purpose I will now draw on the theoretical base of Developmental Transformations (Johnson, 2009) which, as an entirely improvisational method, relies on the study of surprise, to see whether it can help illuminate this core element of Self-Rev.

Developmental Transformations is an arts-based, performative practice in which the client, called a player, spontaneously enacts how they are feeling and thinking with a therapist, called a playor, and other players if in a group format. This practice can occur in any arts modality, though DvT was created within a drama therapy context. DvT is based on *Instability Theory*, which relies primarily on Buddhist, existentialist, and postmodern influences (Johnson, 2013). The primary axiom of Instability Theory is that *experience is nonrepeating*. Experience of each and every present moment is completely new, because each and every present moment has never been before. This moment... this moment... this moment. Everything changes, as Heraclitus (2003) observed long ago: 'One cannot step into the same river twice.' Yet this description does not seem to match our experience, which is that each moment seems to be largely a combination of other moments and things: I am David, again, waking up and brushing my teeth, again, and driving my Chevy to work, again, and sitting in that same room in the same meeting, again, on May 8, again. Life seems largely a repetition, as noted (also) long ago in Ecclesiastes 1:9: 'there is nothing new under the sun.' Indeed, we are accustomed to innumerable repeating forms: letters, words, numbers, sentences, objects, places, people, stories. These representations of experience (representations) are at heart language. We give form to infinity by arbitrarily naming points on a line with repeating numerals (which we made up); we describe the universe in English by using 26 scribbles/letters (which we made up). By agreeing on sets of repeating forms, we can effectively communicate with each other; in addition, we can stabilize our experience of this potentially overwhelming world. Thus, lived experience appears to be a combination of repeating and nonrepeating elements. Desires for stability inevitably deny, minimize, or even eliminate awareness of the non-repeating elements, though this risks experiencing life as a never-ending repetition, as rote, as dead. (Dead relationships or marriages are characterized by the couple focusing on what is the same rather than what is new.) Instability theory claims however that the nonrepeating element can never be eliminated from an experience, and that learning how to notice and feel it, is essential to being in the moment, in becoming (Johnson, 2013). The animation of a person, a performance, or a relationship is therefore dependent upon the unstable dance between repeating and nonrepeating elements, and the degree to which the parties notice and appreciate what is new and emergent. This requires the courage to face the unknown and to adapt to a new demand, to experience in life 'that fragile, fluctuating center which forms never reach' (Artaud, 1958, p. 13).

The direct result of this primary axiom is what is called the *prime discrepancy*: that representations of experience are not the same as experience. That is, the map of the world is not the world; our descriptions of how we feel are not how we feel. This discrepancy is the source of our existential instability, in its forms of suffering and anxiety, but also in its forms of development, hope, and becoming. Representations of experience (which include all language, as well as performance) are therefore unstable, because they can never completely and accurately capture our experience of the present moment. Take, for example, spoken language, which consists of a set of words from a particular language, such as, 'Hi, sweetheart, I think that haircut looks marvelous on you!' These words are the repeating forms that constitute a complete, accurate, and unambiguous sentence in English. Yet when someone speaks these lines, they use many variations of intonation, speed, volume, cadence, and facial and postural inflections, which give the same sentence many different meanings. These intonations and variations are spontaneously created; they are inherently ambiguous and there is no dictionary that lists them. They can never be repeated in exactly the same way because as soon as you say the phrase once, you feel slightly different. They communicate a person's desires, associations, doubts, and beliefs outside and around what the defined word forms can communicate. Thus, with your partner, you must use the word 'love' often, but it is how you say it that lets your partner know if you do in fact feel love for them at that moment. And likewise, in the theatre, you must use the scripted lines, but it is how you say them that brings the characters to life for the audience, and constitutes good acting.

Not only is language incomplete, but language actually causes the absence that destabilizes it, a deep irony. Imagine if you could experience all the sounds, colors, textures, smells, and stimuli available to you at one moment, without dividing these up into forms or objects or things. At that moment Being would be full: all is here, nothing is missing, 'this is.' Such is the state of emptiness, of nirvana, of oneness. Now imagine organizing one part of that swirl of stimuli into an object, say 'mommy,' with its particular shape, color, smell, size, and detail, and now with its name. Language, representation, has acted to create a piece of the world. However, as soon as this combination of stimuli moves and disappears (for example, when I turn my head or she exits the room), mommy is 'gone.' Then she returns, and I have a feeling about her, I am happy, and then she is gone again, and I feel sadness and longing. I call out to have her come back! And she does, or she does not. Where has she gone? A new entity is now created: *elsewhere*. And each time I learn the name of a new combination of elements, I simultaneously add to my knowledge of, and attachment to, the world, and am thrown into a world of loss, of absence, of 'elsewheres,' and of suffering. Ironically, the nonrepeating elements can never disappear, for they are always here right now, and only now. Their only chance of survival is to become labeled by language, and therefore to become repeating, and enter the tumble of here-and-gone like all the rest. We are faced with another deep irony: to survive is to be repeatable, to come and then to go, to be born and then to die. Only the present is eternal, though ever-changing. This is a meaning of the story of Adam and Eve and the tree of knowledge: To know is to be separated from Eden.

It turns out, however, that this elsewhere—the capacity of repeating forms to disappear—becomes the basis of all other elsewheres that will populate our human experience, including 'mental imagery,' 'mind,' 'imagination,' 'past and future,' 'world,' and most profoundly 'others.' They contain all the things we have experienced and which are no longer in our physical presence. These elsewheres are the ephemeral, liminal, partial, misty spaces that are constructed out of the dynamics among the basic instabilities. They are the foundations of the transitional and ambiguous territories of intimacy, play, magic, dream, creativity, art, and theatre. In them, new arrangements and combinations are created and played with, which will become the source of the new discoveries, surprises, and insights that come to us in the working through process of the Self-Rev.

I propose that the experience of surprise is the result of a disruption in the experience of repeating forms by a nonrepeating element: the arrival of the unexpected from elsewhere. We think something is true or real or here and suddenly, it's not (or at least not entirely)! Surprise is the awareness of the prime discrepancy; it is the reaction to the simultaneous experience of repeating and nonrepeating elements, of a given to the spontaneous. It is the realization that the way I am perceiving the world is not the world.

Instability theory proposes that there are *three primary affects of surprise*—emotional reactions that tell us that a person is surprised. First, if the eruption of the new is perceived to be positive or gratifying, the affect is *delight*! If the new element is perceived to be negative or threatening, the affect will be *alarm*! And if the new element is balanced in terms of positive and negative aspects, the affect will be *awe*! The physical form of these affects are remarkably similar: usually an open mouth and eyes with a raising of the chest and outstretching of the arms. Only small nuances in the shaping of the mouth and movement of the head separate these affective behaviors.

If we are to understand the elements of surprise within a theatrical performance, the observation of repeating and nonrepeating forms will be essential, as well as noting the emergence of the primary affects. Thus instability theory predicts that for a Self-Rev performance to elicit discovery in the moment, the actor must become aware of the nonrepeating element within a repeating structure (the script and rehearsed actions), and experience an affect of surprise. It is important to emphasize that it is the actor who experiences this surprise (not acting as if their character were surprised), and that this spontaneous reaction is communicated to the audience. This may be essentially the same question as: How does an actor bring life to rehearsed actions?—which has been the preoccupation of theatre artists for over a century. How does one pretend to be living in the moment? How does the actor create the illusion of presence, that is, the 'as if'?

THE ROLE OF DISCREPANCY IN METHODS OF ACTING

The project of reliably training actors to bring life to their characters has not been a theoretical question: acting is a difficult skill and directors are constantly presented with bad acting. Though each of the major methods of acting training is justified by the unique perspective of its founder, instability theory predicts that each method must in some way recreate the fundamental condition of the prime discrepancy. Good acting must therefore be the simultaneous presentation of repeating and nonrepeating elements to the audience. Since the script and blocking are the repeating forms, something else must be enacted simultaneously, and this something else must have never been before and therefore arise from a source other than the script or play, each time the play is performed. An examination of major acting theories reveals that each one results in a state of discrepancy in the actor's behavior.

In Stanislavski's (1936) *affective memory method,* for example, actors are trained to recall a personal memory that evokes a feeling similar to that required in their character. The intent is to make emotions more easily available to the actor at particular moments of the play. However, this approach requires a twofold consciousness in the actor: that of the character and that of one's own personal past. At the moment in question, the actor continues to say his/her lines but shifts attention to their personal memory and its emotive qualities. The audience perceives this dual focus, in which the actor is partly not in role, which gives the performance its power and authenticity. Thus a discrepancy is enacted.

Grotowski (1968) experimented with whether the actor needed to remember an actual personal memory, when in *The Constant Prince,* he asked Richard Ciezlak to imagine an entirely different scenario while playing the lead character. Throughout the play, as Ciezlak was enacting his character and speaking the lines from the script, he was imagining the unfolding a completely different story. The audience must have perceived the actor's dual focus, his partly not being present in the given story, his absence, which made the performance electric. Again, the essential condition is to instill a state of discrepancy in the actor. Similarly, Bertolt Brecht's (1977) *alienation effect* and Michael Chekhov's (1953) *psychological gesture* also produce multilayered, discrepant behaviors within the actor, either by having the actor place themselves psychologically outside their character (Brecht), or by developing an abstract, personal gesture/symbol of the character that is contained within the actor (Chekhov).

Meisner's *repetition exercise* is the most clearly developed method of playing with repeating and nonrepeating forms (Meisner & Longwell, 1987). No one was more aware than Meisner of the tension between repetition and impulse (nonrepeating elements). In the repetition exercise, actors interact while repeating the same lines over and over again. Usually the lines make reference to the behavior of the other actor, such as 'You seem unhappy with me right now.' Actors are asked to say the line based on how the other person is actually behaving in the moment, and therefore learn how to read the nonrepeating elements in the other. Inevitably, they find that different impulses arise that shift and transform the deliverance of the line, in response to the other actor's behavior. The actor is therefore trained to place their attention on these emerging impulses both in themselves and the other, rather than the repeated lines. The goal is to be truthful not to the script, but to the lived moment, and therefore 'to live truthfully under imaginary circumstances.' The technique restrains actors from attempting to 'be' their character (as in the Method), which thereby reduces the discrepancy between behaving naturally and the imaginary situation of the play.

Many theatre directors use *improvisational methods* to help actors enliven their performances: they have them go through the play at double speed, in a different language, as animals, with roles reversed, etc. Improvisation is driven by new or unexpected elements. The fundamental requirement of improvisation, to say 'yes' to these nonrepeating elements instead of 'blocking an offer,' is the source of animation, fun, and excitement of improv (Johnstone, 1987). To block an offer is to refuse surprise. All these exercises introduce discrepant associations and feelings in the actor, which later help bring nuances into their performance, enlivening the script and evoking a feeling of presence.

Discrepancy is therefore critical to good acting, and the reason is that real people are discrepant. Playing only those actions that are consistent with a particular role leads to acting that is flat, rote, and one-dimensional, being a narrow replay of the script. It is like the difference between a natural voice and a computer-generated one. Bad acting is similar to Sartre's (1966) concept of *bad faith*, where the person acts only in a manner consistent with their social role: I am a waiter, therefore I will move like a waiter, I will speak like a waiter. This is bad faith because the person violates the essential condition of human reality as a 'being which is what it is not, and which is not what it is' (p. 58). We are more than the map of ourselves; the actor must play more than what the script lays out. The audience is looking for signs of both the scripted role and a living, spontaneous person.

THE MOMENT OF WORKING THROUGH DURING SELF-REV PERFORMANCE

If good acting is to be able to infuse one's character with the truthfulness and spontaneity of oneself, how can that be done when one's character is oneself, as it is in Self-Rev?! What is the source of discrepancy between myself and my portrayal of myself?

In a Self-Rev, the actor plays a character that is him/herself. It is crucial to recognize that this representation of self is not the self. Since the characterization has been rehearsed, it is a repeating form and therefore cannot fully be the person. Thus it is possible to imagine another actor learning the script and performing the role (though the performance would no longer be a Self-Rev). *The power of Self-Rev is derived wholly from the reality that the actor is playing him/herself, and that there is nevertheless a discrepancy between the actor and the dramatic character being played.*

A unique situation exists: the character is the actor, so the distance between the two may seem to collapse in the audience's mind. As the character being portrayed follows the rehearsed lines and actions, the actor is there, experiencing the moment for the first time. In a regular performance where the actor is playing a role that is not themselves, the actor's personal feelings in the moment are intended to enhance the aliveness of the acting, but are not intended to be identified to the audience as the actor's feelings. The actor enacts discrepant elements but in order for these to be attributed to the character; in contrast, the Self-Rev actor enacts discrepant elements that are not cloaked in this way, but are purposefully revealed as belonging to the actor him/herself.

This works because in a Self-Rev performance the audience cares about the story of the actor, but they care even more about the actor. Thus, while revealing how an actor feels in a regular drama will interfere with the purpose of the play, in a Self-Rev what the actor is going through *is* the play. When the audience sees it happening in the moment, it is even more electrifying for them. Powerful moments of Self-Rev occur when the audience sees the actor's vulnerability, fear, and courage in the moment, not unlike the excitement generated when an acrobat wobbles on the high wire.

This suggests that moments of working through occur at times when the rehearsed flow is interrupted, or interfered with by an emotional reaction of the actor, and *where the actor integrates that response into the flow of the performance*. Examples of this might include: (1) the actor interrupts the flow of performance with a reaction, or looks out at the audience with an affect of surprise, or shows an affect not consistent with that moment in the play; (2) the actor makes an actual out of role comment about their feelings about the performance, or spontaneously asks an audience member to comment or react; (3) the actor plays out divergent possible responses to an issue (as part of the rehearsed play) but in performing them shows feelings that are obviously being experienced in the moment. In all these cases, the audience will be signaled that the actor is having feelings or thoughts discrepant from the expected, rehearsed actions of the performance.

In these critical moments, both actor and audience will be thrown into a state of instability, simultaneously experiencing reality and imagination, play and presence, pain and joy. The characteristics of instability, ambiguity, and uncertainty create the dramatic tension inherent in any moment of good theatre: the dance of the present and elsewhere, of form and impulse. This formulation is very similar to the concept of the *performative* discussed by Gideon Zehavi in Chapter 11.

In a Self-Rev performance, in these moments of working through, the real person pokes through the mask of the performance of self: in this way the self is revealed. The form has been well-named. Only by 'self' what is meant is the 'self in this moment' in its nonrepeating form, not the 'self of the persona and biographical story.' What the audience experiences is not the actor's character, but the actor him/herself, signaling through the flames, vulnerable, at risk.

The audience will be impacted in a similar manner in these moments of working through, for they too care whether the actor survives; they too are affected if the actor transforms himself through the healing process. In these moments, the audience's roles will become split: they will remain audience to the play, and also become acutely aware of being support-ers of the actor. The stakes of these two roles are vastly different. This situation is not unlike those moments when parents attend a dance or theatrical performance of their children: often they hardly notice the play, as they are completely engaged in walking with their child through each moment they are on stage. Imagine how a parent would feel if that child, in the middle of their performance, looked out at them and communi-cated a feeling in the moment about being on stage, positive or nega-tive? Most parents' hearts would leap out of their chest (if they didn't feel like leaping out of their chairs!). They would then have to restrain that impulse. Similarly in Self-Rev: the audience's reactions as real friends/family may be as strong, but must be suppressed due to the demands of being an audience member and not disrupting the performance. Rather than a problem, this is the parallel process in the audience of working through in the actor, and therefore is essential. For the essence of working through is confronting this question: *'Despite what I have lived through, and how I have adapted to its consequences, how do I want to live my life today and in the future? To what degree do I want to carry forward my past into the present?'* If there were to be an audience debriefing after a Self-Rev (which I strongly recommend), this is the crucial experience to examine and share: how did it feel to be both audience and friend/family? It is a cruel irony that with our intimates we must often refrain from sharing our observations of their struggles, of their performances of themselves, out of respect for them. After they go on in great detail about an issue they have repeatedly struggled with, for years, we simply look them deeply in their eyes, and smile lovingly. This is the contact we make with them as present beings, outside and around all the persona, history, issues, roles, and language of self. This is why we can love them though they may irri-tate us. Thus in the successful Self-Rev, the actor may be able to make this type of pure, if transient, contact with the audience: creating an opening in the dramatic form to peek out at the audience, who reply, 'regardless of the performance of the story, we love you anyway, always.' In the end, then, Self Rev may not be about a performance as much as it is about the revelation of a person in the present moment.

CONCLUSION

The self-revelatory performance process can indeed find a primary source of Otherness within the performance itself, by the actor revealing spontaneous reactions to the issues presented in the play, so that the actor–audience interaction is infused in a double manner by the real and imaginal elements of this dramatic encounter. The true Self-Rev is never a presentation of a therapeutic process already concluded, but rather of a story interrupted by the unscripted, nonrepeating, surprising experience of the actor who at that moment is unsure of himself, and uncertain of the safety or integrity of his very being. Crucially, the actor both opens themselves to the emergence of these feelings in the moment, and simultaneously integrates them into the flow of the performance. The working through process during a performance necessarily throws the audience out of its role as audience, into its real relationships with the actor, in a state of care for them. An unstable state of imbalance between repeating and nonrepeating elements of being occurs, a state of presence sought in any good theatre and in any good therapy.

REFERENCES

Artaud, A. (1958). *The theatre and its double.* New York: Grove Press.

Brecht, B. (1977). *Brecht on theatre: The development of an aesthetic* (13th ed.). New York: Hill & Wang.

Chekhov, M. (1953). *To the actor: On the technique of acting.* New York: Harper & Brothers.

Emunah, R. (2015). Self-revelatory performance: A form of drama therapy and theater. *Drama Therapy Review, 1*(1), 71–85.

Grotowski, J. (1968). *Towards a poor theatre.* New York: Methuen.

Heraclitus (2003). *Fragments.* New York: Penguin Classics.

Johnson, D. (2009). Developmental transformations. In D. Johnson & R. Emunah (Eds.), *Current approaches in drama therapy* (pp. 89–116). Springfield, IL: Charles C. Thomas.

Johnson, D. (2013). Text for Practitioners II. New Haven, CT: Institute for Developmental Transformations. Available at www.developmentaltransformations.com

Johnstone, K. (1987). *Impro: Improvisation for the theatre.* New York: Routledge.

Koestler, A. (1964). *The act of creation.* London: Penguin.

Meisner, S., & Longwell, D. (1987). *Sanford Meisner on acting.* New York: Random House.

Sartre, J. P. (1969). *Being and nothingness.* New York: Methuen.

Stanislavski, C. (1936). *An actor prepares.* New York: Theatre Arts Books.

CHAPTER 6

Relational Aesthetics in the Performance of Personal Story

Nisha Sajnani

Performing one's life on stage in drama therapy involves giving aesthetic expression to lived experience in the service of healing for both actors and audiences. Within the field of drama therapy, there are several unique genres or approaches to the performance of personal story, including *self-revelatory, autobiographical,* and *autoethnographic* theater to name a few (Emunah, 1994, 2015; Harnden, 2014; Sajnani, 2012). While these form differ from one another, they all involve an interlacing of clinical efficacy and artistic accomplishment or what I have referred to elsewhere as *relational aesthetics* (Sajnani, 2012). This chapter expands upon this concept from an interdisciplinary perspective in order to advance a poetics of performance in drama therapy in which ethics and aesthetics are seen not as competing objectives rather than contiguous processes that are mutually supportive. In particular, I will focus on how viewing the performance of personal story through the prism of relational aesthetics may contribute to our understandings of the self, healing, artistry, ethics, and audience in this practice.

N. Sajnani, PhD, RDT-BCT (✉)
Lesley University, Cambridge, MA, USA

New York University, New York, NY, USA

University of Melbourne, Melbourne, Australia
e-mail: nishasajnani75@gmail.com

© The Author(s) 2016   85
S. Pendzik et al. (eds.), *The Self in Performance*,
DOI 10.1057/978-1-137-53593-1_6

A Relational View of the Self and Healing

The majority of drama therapists espouse a relational view of the self whether we privilege the intentional invocation and interrelation of intra-psychic and interpersonal roles (Landy, 2009) or the 'continuous transformation of embodied encounters in a playspace' (Johnson, 2014, p. 38). Understandings of the self, both our own and our clients', influence therapeutic and aesthetic choices. If, per Landy's *Role Theory* (2009), we understand the self as a series of roles and the purpose of therapy as being about tolerating ambiguity, contradiction and gaining perspective, it would follow that the performance may involve the embodiment of 'parts of the self' or 'taking on the roles of others' (Emunah, 2015, p. 75). If, per Johnson's theory of *Developmental Transformations* (2009), we understand the self or being as a presence that, in an effort to cope with ever-changing experience, becomes obstructed by impulses expressed as behaviors designed to control one's environment, the purpose of therapy and the purpose of performance might become about strengthening one's capacity to tolerate change by placing one's attention on the newness of the present moment. While these approaches differ, both 'emphasize connection and interconnectedness as formative and forming to the individual, those around them and the contexts they live in' (Jones, 2007, p. 230). The drama therapist's skilled use of symbolic communication and metaphor to find aesthetic distance (Bullough, 1912; Landy, 1983; Scheff, 1981) along with other core processes such as play, transformation, embodiment, projection, and witnessing (Jones, 2007) serve to heighten one's experience of connectedness to self and to other.

This understanding of how an intentional aesthetic engagement facilitates relationship reflects somewhat recent trends in contemporary performance art that, in turn, may illuminate and expand aspects of our practice. Nicolas Bourriard (1998) first coined the term *relational aesthetics* to describe the cultural production of artists in the 1990s whose art reflected a changing psychological landscape emerging from a growing interest and engagement with the internet and its capacities to foster social networks (Sajnani, 2012). According to Bourriard, relational aesthetics encompasses 'a set of artistic practices which take, as their theoretical and practical point of departure, the whole of human relations and their social context, rather than an independent and private space' (1998, p. 113). Relational art reflects and prompts interconnections between people, groups, and systems by creating a delineated social circumstance, or what Bourriard referred to as a 'proposal to live in a shared world' (1998, p. 154), in which 'the moment of shared communication is the realization of the art-work' (Chayka, 2011, p. 1).

The therapeutic benefit of performing personal story in drama therapy is derived, in part, from its capacity to create a shared world in which performers find a means to invite their audiences to witness those parts of themselves that 'have been hidden from public domain [and] that have been kept secret' (Emunah, 1994, p. 251), or to transcend stigmatiz-ing identities (Emunah & Johnson, 1983; Orkibi, Bar, & Eliakim, 2014; Sajnani, 2012; Snow, 2009). We assume that this is accomplished, in part, by elevating lived experience onto what Susana Pendzik has referred to as a *sacred space* (1994) or what David Read Johnson has referred to as the *playspace* (2009) where the 'macrocosm of the world can be represented... and invested with extreme significance' (Bailey, 2009, p. 374) and where one can be witnessed by a supportive audience. However, a considerable challenge lies in how to create a shared world that is accessible to both the actor/person served and the audience (Emunah, 1994, 2015). In other words, the performance of personal story in drama therapy must reflect the unique concerns of the performer(s) and facilitate one's capacity to remain present but it must also resonate with audiences in order to realize its relational purpose.

A RELATIONAL VIEW OF ART

Relational art critic Chakya (2011) states that the primary 'task of the artist is to become a conduit for social experience' (p. 1). Of course, in the context of writing or performing personal story, the artist or actor seldom works alone. Rather, artistry unfolds from those involved in what Phillipe Lejeune has referred to as *le pacte autobiographique* (the autobio-graphical pact) which includes the 'the writer, the narrated subject (which includes the narrator and the character) and the reader (Lejeune cited in Grace, 2003, p. 5). In the context of performing personal story in drama therapy, this pact might include the participant, drama therapist, director, playwright, members of the audience, and the sponsoring agency or institution (Hodermarska, Landy, Dintino, Mowers, & Sajnani, 2015; Sajnani, 2010, 2012). Thus, the artistic task of creating a shared world or a conduit for relational experience arises from the interplay between all of those involved.

This represents a shift from what applied theater theorist Edward Little (2005) has referred to as 'classical aesthetics' which emphasizes 'the skills and accomplishments of the author, director, designer, and actor-in-role, seeks universality in representation, and advocates a clear aesthetic separation between practices involving "art" and the participatory life of a community' (p. 2). Rather, Little asserts that a relational aesthetic implies that artistic 'vision, relevance, interpretation, and authenticity proceed from localized cultural expression that is rooted in a communal sense of utility, participation in art and public life, and a "grass-roots-up" inspired philosophy of cultural democracy' (p. 1). Artistic vision, quality, originality, accuracy, relevance, and insight are criteria directly connected to a relational process through which artistic choices are made from the development of a character, to the writing of a script, to the staging of a scene. Therefore, the strength of the process leading to the stage is integral to the performance of personal story in drama therapy.

On the surface, these ideas reflect common practice in drama therapy in that drama therapists often claim to follow the lead of the person served (Cassidy, Turnbull, & Gumley, 2014). Drama therapists work together with participants to find 'forms, texts, images, and metaphors for inner feeling states' (Harnden, 2014, p. 148). In the context of performance, a drama therapist may aid another to organize and 'encapsulate experiences in the form of a story' towards increased emotional regulation and insight amongst other social, emotional, cognitive, and behavioral goals (Bailey, 2009, p. 374). In addition to the drama therapist, a playwright or director may be engaged to strengthen the artistry of the performance which, in turn, presents the audience with a carefully crafted invitation to enter into the world of the performer (Bailey, 2009; Emunah, 1994, 2015). Each one plays a role in bringing the struggles and conflicts faced by the person served to the stage.

Yet, when it comes to the final performance, many performances adopt the Aristotelian prescription of a protagonist-centered drama (Alker, 2015). Therefore, the representation of individuals claiming their independence through performance, while courageous and potentially empowering obscures the interdependence of the artist, audience, and other authorizing agents. The therapist, for example, seldom takes the stage—though there have been notable and daring exceptions (Kilgannon, 2014; Sajnani, 2012). The rationale here is that, if the stage offers a heightened experience of self and other, there may be therapeutic benefit to having the therapist and client explore their relationship within a performative frame. Granted, this would need to be carefully considered with the client and some elements of the play may need to remain static (e.g. the staging, the script) to permit a playful, performative exploration between therapist and client. A relational aesthetic calls up ways of making relationships transparent thus transforming singular accounts of lived experience into an acknowledgement of one's interdependence within a co-constructed, dynamic, living system (see Hodermarska et al. in this book). Such an approach might also raise useful questions about ownership and the challenges of sharing authority between clients, directors, drama therapists, and the needs and goals of the agency or sponsoring institution.

A RELATIONAL VIEW OF ETHICS

The interplay of the actor, drama therapist, director, playwright and others (e.g. students, auxiliaries, partners, children, etc.) involved in the development of a performance featuring personal story involves a negotiation. Another way to think about this negotiation is as an ethical process in which choices are given due consideration. As stated by relational ethics scholar, Mark Pharoah (2009), 'the question is not, what behavior is right, but what […] makes it right?' (p. 1). A relational ethic does not presume a singular moral choice or a choice determined by external moral standards but places emphasis on the needs, emotions, concepts, relationships, and context in which choices are made. Carolyn Ellis (2007), in a discussion about auto/ethnography and auto/ethnographic research, argues that 'relational ethics requires researchers to act from our hearts and minds, acknowledge our interpersonal bonds to others, and take responsibility for actions and their consequences' (p. 3). Personal stories arise from a social context in which our spouses, partners, children, friends, neighbors, and/or colleagues may be implicated (Ellis, Adams, & Bochner, 2011; Sajnani, 2004).

In drama therapy, a concept that reflects a relational understanding of ethics is Johnson's articulation of *mutuality*, which he defines as an agreement between those involved (2009, p. 93). This agreement, at least in the context of Johnson's articulation of Developmental Transformations, is not forged and forgotten at the beginning of the process but revisited as needed along the way. This developmental, organic, and relational approach to consent and choice-making is highly relevant to a discussion of relational aesthetics in the context of performing personal story and points to the need for transparent and ongoing conversations between clients/actors and the people in their lives who are implicated and who may witness the performance and between those involved in making therapeutic and aesthetic choices as discussed in an earlier section.

A Relational View of the Audience

Another area where a relational aesthetic perspective may be useful to consider is in our conception of the audience. In performance-oriented drama therapy, those performing take a risk to reveal themselves to a chosen audience. Drama therapists embrace a relational perspective in that there is consideration given to who is in the audience and what their relationships are to those performing. Making decisions about who will bear witness to the performance is an important part of what we consider to be healing in this practice (Bailey, 2009). However, as I have argued previously, the audience in drama therapy is often described as a monolith and often given a very limited role (Sajnani, 2010, 2012).

In Bourriard's relational art, the audience is not sedentary or hidden in the dark as is often the case in mainstream theater and in the majority of performances featuring personal story. Rather, audience members are individuals who move, interact, and have ideas and impulses of their own that arise in the present moment (Chakya, 2011). This is an area in which our dramaturgy might benefit from the risks taken in contemporary and feminist performance art. For example, in 2010, Serbian artist Marina Abramović performed a piece entitled *The Artist is Present* at a retrospective about her work at the Museum of Modern Art in New York. As is characteristic of her work, she created an opportunity for audiences to encounter her body. In this piece, she sat at a table across from 1565 voluntary spectators for a total of 736 hours and 30 minutes and, over time, observed the poignancy of these encounters:

> What is very new about this performance is that we always perceive the audience as a group, but a group consists of many individuals. In this piece I deal with individuals of that group and it's just a one-to-one relationship. So, when you enter the square of light and you sit on that chair, you're an individual, and as an individual you are kind of isolated. And you're in a very interesting situation because you're observed by the group (the people waiting to sit), you're observed by me, and you're observing me—so it's like triple observation. But then, very soon while you're having this gaze and looking at me, you start having this invert and you start looking at yourself.

So I am just a trigger, I am just a mirror and actually they become aware of their own life, of their own vulnerability, of their own pain, of everything—and that brings the crying. [They are] really crying about their own self, and that is an extremely emotional moment. (Abramović in Stigh & Jackson, 2010, para. 5)

Here the audience is understood as a complex body that informs and interacts with the performer and the performance. Audience members are not uniformly cast as witnesses present only to listen or to see but invited to engage all of their senses in the immediacy of a shared encounter in which all who are present might be transformed. In fact, in a moment reminiscent of Grotowski's *poor theater* (Grotowski, 1968; Johnson, Forrester, Dintino, James, & Schnee, 1996), Abramović chose to remove the table in the middle of her performance. When asked about why, she responded:

Many years ago I was always talking about future art and I was thinking about this idea of how in the future objects should be removed and it should be just the transmission of energy between [artist] and the public. In the end of April I had the man with a wheelchair and in the middle of this piece I realized that I didn't even know he had legs because the table is there, I don't see. So I decided to remove the table and when I removed the table then the piece started having sense to me. I know now that I'm really interested more and more in immaterial art, that removing the table is just this direct connection. And I think that reached the point with the public reaction emotionally the most. I mean, everybody comes there, sits five minutes, and is already in tears, crying. It really removed all the obstacles. (Abramović in Stigh & Jackson, 2010, para. 6)

In another example, Argentinean-born Thai artist Rikrit Tiravanija held a solo show at the 303 gallery in New York during which he cooked Thai food for visitors in a kitchen set up within a gallery, noting that 'it is not what you see that is important but what takes place between people' (Tiravanija in Chakya, 2011, p. 1). By elevating everyday social relations to performance, Tiravanija created an opportunity for the audience to become immersed in his reality while also remaining actively engaged. These two examples, from Abramović and Tiravanija, contribute to what drama therapist Roger Grainger has referred to as 'the therapeusis of the audience' (1996, p. 27) in that, through promenade and immersive staging techniques, the audience is released from their typical constraints. Such performances use smell, touch, place, space, sound, light, and shadow to stimulate the senses, encourage participation, and create a more intimate encounter with another within a carefully considered playspace. As a result, both actors and audiences may experience greater authenticity, empathy, insight, and the possibility of belonging (Furman, 1988; Sajnani, 2012).

Bourriard's articulation of relational aesthetics and the artistic practices that proceed from this notion of relational art have also drawn criticism. For example, Chakya (2011) critiques Tiravanija noting that, while 'the communal experience of cooking and eating the food becomes the object on display', it does so 'under the direction of the artist, who acts as a sort of experience "curator," or maybe "ringmaster" would be a better term' (p. 3). Similarly, critic Hal Foster observed, 'the institution may over-shadow the work that it otherwise highlights: it becomes the spectacle, it collects the cultural capital, and the director-curator becomes the star' (cited in Bishop, 2004, pp. 54–5). Thus, the heightened experience of intimacy and social interaction procured through these events is simulta-neously enabled yet potentially undercut by the fact that they are focused uniquely on the effort of the independent artist as star and by the fact that they have been sanctioned by invisible authorities.

This idea is connected to an earlier point about acknowledging the interdependence and the influence of the relationships that give rise to the self in performance. It also draws attention to which relationships may not be represented when performing personal story. For example, those who might disagree with the assertions and claims made by per-formers are generally not invited to bear witness. Thus, the social and familial relationships that present a challenge to the individual in everyday life—those relationships which may give rise to shame and stigma—remain hidden and avoid critique. The institutions that may benefit from preserv-ing a distinction between the healthy and the mentally ill often remain untouched. For example, a city that funds the work of a local group of adults with physical disabilities may enable them to stage a performance based on their lived experience but is not necessarily held accountable to any changes concerning physical access. In fact, the city may be lauded for its progressive policies. A family that keeps the secret of a daughter's sexual abuse may not necessarily be invited to witness or, if present, necessarily be moved to accommodate the revelations shared by the daughter/per-former. Granted, these kinds of material changes are not usually the main objective in therapeutic processes in which the goal is for one person to attend to the ways in which relational conflicts have resulted in internalized distress. However, these realities ask us to consider the limits of performing personal story and our notions of healing (Sajnani, 2013).

Summary

The concept of *relational aesthetics* provides a language with which to describe the intertwining of psychological and aesthetic aims in the context of performance in drama therapy. Being able to remain in relationship, in connection to oneself and to others amidst and beyond distressing experiences, is assumed here to be an important part of what contributes to healing and to resilience. In our practice, the use of movement, touch, sound, light, shadow, smell, character, role, story, and place, for example, stimulate the senses thus heightening exploration within the therapeutic relationship. In this chapter, I have focused on the value of this concept with regard to the performance of personal story. To this end, I presented and discussed the importance of a relational lens in how drama therapists conceive of the self, healing, artistry, ethics, and the audience. Relational aesthetics privilege the relationships that give rise to and result from the aesthetic performance of personal story. I have also highlighted how the concept of relational aesthetics within the related fields of feminist performance art and applied theater may expand how drama therapists grapple with notions of artistic quality, consent, choice-making, and ownership over the resulting product. While not wanting to be prescriptive, these ideas also highlight the possibilities inherent in participatory, interactive, and immersive staging and also question the limits of performing personal story.

References

Alker, G. (2015). A feminist rethinking of drama therapy: The role of aesthetics and audience in *Cancer as Change Maker*. *Drama Therapy Review, 1*(2), 187–199.

Bailey, S. (2009). Performance in drama therapy. In D. R. Johnson & R. Emunah (Eds.), *Current approaches in drama therapy* (pp. 374–389). Springfield, IL: Charles C. Thomas.

Bishop, C. (2004). Antagonism and relational aesthetics. *October, 110*, 51–59.

Bourriard, N. (1998). *Relational aesthetics.* Dijon, France: Les Presses du Reel.

Bullough, E. (1912). Psychical distance as a factor in art and an aesthetic principle. *British Journal of Psychology, 5*(2), 87–118.

Cassidy, S., Turnbull, S., & Gumley, A. (2014). Exploring core processes facilitating therapeutic change in dramatherapy: A grounded theory analysis of published case studies. *Arts in Psychotherapy, 41*, 353–365.

Chakya, K. (2011). WTF is… Relational Aesthetics?. Accessed January 5, 2015, from http://hyperallergic.com/18426/wtf-is-relational-aesthetics/

Ellis, C. (2007). Telling secrets, revealing lives: Relational ethics in research with intimate others. *Qualitative Inquiry, 13*(1), 3–29.

Ellis, C., Adams, T. E., & Bochner, A. P. (2011). Autoethnography: An overview. *Forum Qualitative Sozialforschung/Forum: Qualitative Social Research, 12*(1). Accessed August 1, 2015, from http://nbn-resolving.de/urn:nbn:de:0114-fqs 1101108

Emunah, R. (1994). *Acting for real: Drama therapy process, technique, and performance.* New York: Brunner-Mazel.

Emunah, R. (2015). Self-revelatory performance: A form of drama therapy and theatre. *Drama Therapy Review, 1*(1), 71–85.

Emunah, R., & Johnson, D. R. (1983). The impact of theatrical performances on the self-images of psychiatric patients. *Arts in Psychotherapy, 10*(4), 233–239.

Furman, L. (1988). Theatre as therapy: The distancing affect applied to audience. *Arts in Psychotherapy, 15*(3), 245–249.

Grace, S. (2003). *Performing the auto/biographical pact: Towards a theory of identity in performance.* Accessed January 5, 2015, from http://www.english.ubc.ca/faculty/grace/thtr_ab.htm

Grainger, R. (1996). The therapeusis of the audience. *Dramatherapy: Journal of British Association of Dramatherapists, 18*(1), 27–31.

Grotowski, J. (1968). *Towards a poor theatre.* New York: Simon & Schuster.

Harnden, B. (2014). You arrive: Trauma performed and transformed. In N. Sajnani & D. R. Johnson (Eds.), *Trauma-informed dramatherapy: Transforming clinics, classrooms, and communities* (pp. 122–151). Springfield, IL: Charles C. Thomas.

Hodermarska, M., Landy, R., Dintino, C., Mowers, D., & Sajnani, N. (2015). As performance: Ethical and aesthetic considerations for therapeutic theater. *Drama Therapy Review, 1*(2), 173–186.

Jones, P. (2007). *Drama as therapy: Theory, practice and research* (2nd ed.). London: Routledge.

Johnson, D. R. (2009). Developmental transformations: Towards the body as presence. In D. R. Johnson & R. Emunah (Eds.), *Current approaches in drama therapy* (pp. 89–116). Springfield, IL: Charles C. Thomas.

Johnson, D. R., Forrester, A., Dintino, C., James, M., & Schnee, G. (1996). Towards a poor drama therapy. *Arts in Psychotherapy., 23*(4), 293–306.

Kilgannon, C. (2014). Therapist and patient share a theater of hurt. Accessed January 5, 2015, from http://www.nytimes.com/2014/11/06/nyregion/therapist-and-patient-share-a-theater-of-hurt.html?_r=0

Landy, R. (1983). The use of distancing in drama therapy. *Arts in Psychotherapy,* *10*(2), 175–185.

Landy, R. (2009). Role theory and the role method of drama therapy. In D. R. Johnson & R. Emunah (Eds.), *Current approaches in drama therapy* (pp. 65–88). Springfield, IL: Charles C. Thomas.

Little, E. (2005). Towards an aesthetic of community-based theatre part II: Avoiding the missionary position. Accessed January 5, 2015, from https://www.yumpu.com/en/document/view/6510721/directors-community-engaged-theatre-in-canada

Orkibi, H., Bar, N., & Eliakim, I. (2014). The effect of drama-based group therapy on aspects of mental illness and stigma. *Arts in Psychotherapy,* *40*(4), 458–466.

Pendzik, S. (1994). The theatre stage and the sacred space: A comparison. *Arts in Psychotherapy,* *21*(1), 25–35.

Pharoah, M. (2009). *Phronesis: The general theory of relational ethics.* Accessed January 5, 2015, from http://homepage.ntlworld.com/m.pharoah/gtre.html

Sajnani, N. (2004). Strategic narratives: The embodiment of minority discourse in biographical performance praxis. *Canadian Theatre Review,* *117*, 33–37.

Sajnani, N. (2010). *Permeable boundaries: Towards a critical, collaborative performance pedagogy.* Unpublished doctoral dissertation. Montreal: Concordia University.

Sajnani, N. (2012). The implicated witness: Towards a relational aesthetic in drama therapy. *Dramatherapy: Journal of British Association of Dramatherapists,* *34*(1), 6–21.

Sajnani, N. (2013). The body politic: The relevance of an intersectional framework for therapeutic performance research in drama therapy. *Arts in Psychotherapy,* *40*(4), 382–385.

Scheff, T. J. (1981). The distancing of emotion in psychotherapy. *Psychotherapy: Theory, Research and Practice,* *8*(1), 46–53.

Snow, S. (2009). Ritual/Theatre/Therapy. In D. R. Johnson & R. Emunah (Eds.), *Current approaches in drama therapy* (pp. 117–144). Springfield, IL: Charles C. Thomas.

Stigh, D., & Jackson, Z. (2010). *Marina Abramović: The artist speaks.* Accessed January 5, 2015, from http://www.moma.org/explore/inside_out/2010/06/03/marina-abramovic-the-artist-speaks

CHAPTER 7

Intersubjectivity in Autobiographical Performance in Dramatherapy

Jean-François Jacques

The aim of this chapter is to explore the autobiographical form of therapeutic theatre in dramatherapy as a relational and intersubjective space whereby the embodied encounter of the performer with the spectator (or witness) creates opportunities for mutual transformation. In other words, this chapter aims to investigate the way in which the production of meaning in autobiographical performance in dramatherapy can be described as emerging from relational and embodied dynamics within the shared space of performance. This inquiry is located within a larger research context that investigates the role of the audience in the production of the performance event and of its meaning. The discussion is mainly carried out from a theoretical perspective, bringing together elements of performance studies, dramatherapy, literary studies, phenomenology and intersubjectivity theory. Lastly, this chapter intends to consider the methodological implications for research of the suggested epistemological and conceptual framework.

I understand *autobiographical performance* (AP) as a form of storytelling whereby the performer engages in an act of sharing a moment of autobiographical memory with an audience. Walter Benjamin describes

J.-F. Jacques, MA (✉)
Anglia Ruskin University, Cambridge, UK
e-mail: jefjacques@aol.com

97
S. Pendzik et al. (eds.), *The Self in Performance*,
DOI 10.1057/978-1-137-53593-1_7

storytelling as 'the ability to exchange experiences' (1999, p. 83). In this way, Benjamin situates storytelling in a system of communication and exchange whereby the recounted experience of the storyteller is, in turn, experienced by a listener in the immediacy of their encounter. They find themselves, Benjamin suggests, in the company of one another. This implies a number of different points that are relevant to the argument developed in this chapter. First, storyteller and listener are co-present and need one another to fulfill their roles and intentions. They are mutually dependent in the sense that the recognition of the other enables the fulfillment of one's own position. Secondly, they share a physical intimacy and proximity that differs for instance from the relationship between novelist and reader which is characterized by spatial and temporal distance. The storyteller–listener relationship is primarily based on the immediacy of their embodied presence. Finally, the togetherness of their being-with in Heideggerian terms creates a community that can be defined through the poiesis generated in the here-and-now of their encounter.

PERFORMANCE AND ENCOUNTER

Peter Brook (1990) famously identified the presence of an *other* watching as essential for a theatrical event to take place. Grotowski (1991) similarly described theatre as an act of encountering an *other* that he located within the internal structure of the self, the person of the fellow actor or the spectator. Grainger (2005), for his part, writes that 'theatre crystallises an experience of betweenness that is creative of personhood' (p. 8). He describes theatre as a living event based on a meeting between actors and audience, and constitutive of individual identity through the participation in and the sharing of an imaginative experience.

I believe three important points can be inferred from this. The first one is to emphasize the centrality of *alterity* in the phenomenology of theatre whereby the proximity and presence of the other raises questions of ethical importance. 'Artistic creation,' writes Todorov, 'cannot be analysed outside of a theory of alterity' (1984, p. 107). Alterity is envisaged here as a position outside of which the construction of a point of view remains incomplete. The other in its ethical dimension becomes a condition for developing an understanding of a given phenomenon as well as being an agent in the production of its meaning. According to the Russian linguist and philosopher Mikhail Bakhtin, 'our real exterior can be seen and understood only by other people, because they are located outside us in space and because they are *others'* (in italics in the text, 1986, p. 7). In the words of Bakhtin (1990), the other provides an 'excess of seeing' which disputes the view of a self that is able to create its own epistemological and ontological truth. In the context of performance, this reminds us how the theatrical event remains intrinsically dependent on an other, separate yet engaged in a shared moment. An ethics of spectatorship in performance (Fitzpatrick, 2011) considers the ethical implications of that dependence and what it means in terms of responsibility. I understand the notion of responsibility for the other as developed by Levinas (1989) as a responsibility for the presence of an other in performance but also, and maybe more importantly, as a recognition of the way the other shapes the performance event and ultimately the subjectivity of those engaged in it.

The second point follows from recognizing the performance event as a dynamic encounter between performers and audience. The question emerges as to who actually creates the performance and where its meaning is located. Barthes (1977) claimed the 'death of the author' to suggest a hermeneutic of text that is no longer centered on the intention of the author but rather on the domain of experience of the reader. A postmodern view suggests that the meaning of an object resides in the eye of the beholder, or to put it differently, that it results from internal projections including what Rozik (2010) names the 'cultural baggage' or normative culture. Yet the postmodern stance has been challenged by refocusing attention to ways in which meaning emerges from a transaction between a reader and a text (Rosenblatt, 1994) and the generative quality of that transaction producing new texts (Smagorinski, 2001). The role of the reader is acknowledged as an active agent in the production of meaning, echoing views of an already emancipated reader/spectator bringing into the performance space his or her own awareness and history (Rancière, 2011). It suggests a subjectivity of spectatorship that had previously been underestimated in the ways in which it shapes the semantic of performance (Bennett, 1997). It also seriously questions the omnipotence of the text as object of analysis (Heddon, 2008) and shifts attention to performance as a process and space whereby 'theatre meaning results from the interaction between a performance-text and a spectator' (Rozik, 2010, p. 161). Finally, it points towards an intersubjective understanding of meaning in performance whereby performer and spectator are both invested, in Hegelian terms, with their own center of consciousness (Stern, 2002).

The third point concerns the nature of that encounter and the fact that it belongs to a singular order of expression as Merleau-Ponty (1962) would say, based on the body. That embodied encounter between performer and spectator is what gives performance its visceral and physical qualities that can literally touch and move us. Performances, remind Shepherd and Wallis (2004), are embodied events whereby experience is communicated and received through the mobilization of the senses. This embodiment of experience is, as Merleau-Ponty (1962) suggested, a privileged vehicle for phenomenological knowledge. Pelias (2008) amongst others explores the implications of embodied experience and of the body as a site of knowledge, echoing what Meyerhold (Pitches, 2003) had previously investigated under the term *embodied knowledge*. This is to be understood at two distinct levels. First, it recognizes the body as a vehicle of communication imprinted with personal and social history, and the depository of social and power relations. Secondly, it envisages the body as an instrument of human inquiry whereby dominant discourses can be expounded and alternatives imagined. This embodied dimension of knowledge captures some of what Judith Butler (1993) describes as a tension between *discursively constituted and constituting subjects,* a tension that is reflected in AP.

Meaning in Autobiographical Performance in Dramatherapy

Autobiographical performance is characterized by an intimate and embodied encounter between a performer and an audience. It is an act of sharing and offering that would not be possible without the presence of an other who in his/her physicality brings out the visibility of the performer. I now turn to the way in which meaning is produced in AP by linking it more specifically to the role of the witness as envisaged in the dramatherapy literature.

Authors tend to generally agree that performing personal stories play an important role in the way we define ourselves and frame our identity (Rubin, 2007; Wood, 2015). In that regard, the act of performing oneself not only communicates parts of personal history but also creates history. This constructivist and narrative perspective emphasizes the way in which narratives help structure experience and more importantly create it (Bruner, 1986). It supports a view of meaning that is not as much archeological in the sense of finding out old truths, as it is teleological or emerging from the nature of a particular experience associated here with the narrative activity. This has resulted in investigating the ontological implications of the self narrating itself and the links between personal narratives and identity. Most notably, it has contributed to the emergence of the concept of *narrative identity* (McAdams, Josselson, & Lieblich, 2006; McAdams & McLean, 2013). This concept suggests that narratives are vehicles through which the self-reflecting individual develops a sense of internal clarity, meaning and purpose. It is characterized by its causal coherence in bringing together fragments of autobiographical memory in a way that helps structure life experience and as a result creates possibilities for change and healing. Narrative identity finds resonance in the field of narrative therapy which claims a reshaping and reclaiming of individual experience through an exploration of saturated and preferred narratives (Payne, 2006).

What can be objected to here, as Czarniawska (2004) puts it, is that 'we are never sole authors of our own narratives' (p. 5). If narratives contribute to a sense of personal meaning, they also reflect a socially constructed self (Holland, Lachicotte, Skinner, & Cain, 2001) or, to paraphrase Judith Butler, they are storied as much as storying by cause of interpersonal experience, social, cultural, discursive and linguistic practices. Besides, the performance of personal narratives takes place in a particular context. This makes performance a situated practice whose prospect and reality can have liberating but also hindering effects on the performer. In that sense, it seems more accurate to talk about situated stories (McLean, Pasupathi, & Pals, 2007). The question to ask is whether meaning emerges from the simple act of telling and performing stories (and therefore described as endogenous) or whether it emerges as a result of the relational context in which it takes place (and therefore described as exogenous). That question raises further questions of ontological difficulties since it forces us to consider the role of the other in the way we define ourselves and construct our identity.

Jones (2007) links the way meaning is constructed in dramatherapy to the presence of others able to empathize and respond to what is being explored and developed. According to him, others as audience are witnesses to a process, and it is in that interaction that possibilities for meaning emerge. Others therefore become a significant therapeutic factor for change. Jones (2005) distinguishes between witnessing and being witnessed in the therapeutic process, although both carry potential for insight and healing. He identifies layers of witnessing within dramatherapy groups (Jones, 2007) whereby the roles of audience and performer (or observer and participant) are constantly interchanged. He acknowledges how the

performer affects the audience by evoking empathy, resonance or identification, but also, I would suggest, by creating possible dissonance or
distance. He sees how the audience affects the performer by fostering
acceptance, validation or recognition, but also by engendering a possible
sense of persecution or isolation. In other words, the performer–audience relationship equally carries significant beneficial and detrimental
effects. Jones does not place his analysis directly in the context of AP,
focusing rather on the internal and interactive audience within dramatherapy groups. Equally, he does not offer a detailed account of the production of meaning in an interactive context. Nevertheless, he highlights the
dynamic relationships of mutual influence and reciprocity between performers and witnesses and how this engagement actively informs meaning
in dramatherapy.

The relationship to the audience and its role in AP and *self-revelatory
performance* (Self-Rev) has been identified as a significant feature by several authors, albeit with different emphases. Emunah (2015) describes
the reciprocity between performer and spectator based on a dynamic relation of empathy validation, but without elaborating on the details of the
mechanics of that reciprocity. Previously, Emunah (1994) recognized the
role played by the audience in relaying a mutual sense of connectedness
following engagement with the issues presented on stage and resulting
in feelings of shared humanity. Rubin (2007) suggests how the ritual of
being witnessed in performance is essential to personal transformation.
Schrader (1998) shares similar views in a context of part-autobiographical
performances whereby she describes the audience as a necessary condition for healing. Sajnani (2012) adopts a larger perspective and envisages
biographical performance as engaging with the lived reality of audiences
and not solely reflecting the lived experience of those performing. Like
MacKay (1996), she views performance as a political act contributing to a
renewal of social dialogue.

This brings me to two final points. First, it is noteworthy that if Jones
(2007) focuses mainly on the role of the audience within dramatherapy
groups, the studies mentioned above tend to concentrate more on the
relationship between performers and external audience. This adds another
layer of witnessing alongside the context in which the performance practice
takes place. I will come back to this point later by trying to think system-
atically about this in relation to the way meaning is produced. Secondly,
there seems to be an agreement on the function of the audience activat-
ing something on behalf of the performer. This remains quite a complex

process to describe that reminds us that performance is more than per-forming. It is done in front of others whose eyes need borrowing in order to see completion, as in the story of the Three Graeae in the Greek myth of Perseus. The Graeae only had one eye between the three of them, an eye that they needed to share and hold in turns in order to see. Without that eye, they were simply condemned to blindness. In other words, they each needed the eye of the other to be able to see. Pitruzzella (2009) offers a useful contribution here by suggesting how the audience is a source of authorization for performers and how this reflects the funda-mental relationality of theatre. Interestingly, the word authorization origi-nates etymologically from the Latin *auctor*, meaning author. According to Pitruzzella, audience and actors are engaged in a mutual act of authoring. It suggests in my opinion that performance is the spatial expression of a unique relationship based on interdependence and mutuality. This also suggests that performance offers renewed capacities to envisage oneself in dialogue with and in relation to others.

Audience, Meaning and Intersubjectivity

In the field of performance studies, recent contemporary practices have highlighted intersubjective processes that seem relevant to the argument developed in this chapter. It is my intention to investigate which aspects of intersubjective theory might help conceptualize the production of mean-ing in AP.

Writing about autobiography as a performance practice, Heddon (2008) argues vehemently against the self-referential and solipsistic nature of the performed personal narrative by considering its historic roots in feminist theory and practice, and its social function of challenging the dominant politics of representation. Heddon (2013) suggests ways in which AP is primarily dialogic through reflecting a number of transactions amongst which is the relationship between performer and spectator. She provides examples of performance artists such as Tim Miller and Robbie McCauley who shift attention from dialogue with the self (Marranca, 1979) to dia-logue with the other in autobiographical work and its scripting in the performance event (Boenisch, 2010). This recognition of the subjectiv-ity of the other (Fitzpatrick, 2011) in performance is also illustrated in the work of other artists, such as Marina Abramović, that Phelan (2004) describes as an 'experiment in intersubjectivity,' whereby the dependence on the audience is fully acknowledged and the artist intentionally enters into an embodied dialogue with the lived experience of the other. The conceptual artist Sophie Calle, in *Exquisite Pain* (2003), juxtaposes her personal experience of separation and pain with the different, yet similar subjective experiences of others in a way that gradually helps her work through her trauma. In these different artistic practices, the commitment to the story of the other is a condition for new rays of meaning to shine out of one's own experience. This is what Madison (2007) describes, referring to the words of Conquergood (1985), as dialogic performance or the expression of 'the meeting of two subjects whose subjectivities grow and deepen from their mutual encounter' (p. 829).

Intersubjectivity offers a useful conceptual framework to understand the way in which the self of the performer and the spectator dialogically relate in their mutual search for meaning. Intersubjectivity originates in the phenomenological philosophy of Husserl and Heidegger, and has developed into a paradigm that has found applications in the fields of humanistic and existential psychotherapy (Nolan, 2012) and psychoanalysis (Benjamin, 1995). It has provided a framework to describe and understand the interpersonal dynamics of infant and human development, but also the particular processes at play in the therapeutic relationship. My intention here is to situate intersubjectivity in the context of performed autobiographies, examining how it can account for an understanding of the different levels of interaction within the intersubjective space of performance, and how this informs the meaning-making process.

The intersubjective space can be defined as being the expression of mutual and reciprocal exchanges and influences between individualities recognized for having their own center of consciousness. It is a coming together of one mind with another who, says Benjamin, 'can be felt with, yet has a distinct, separate center of feeling and perception' (2004, p. 5). The intersubjective space is not solely the expression of dyadic relationships but also of different levels of *being-in-the-world-with-others* (Cornejo, 2008). As a dialectic expression of a meeting of different subjectivities, it is a window through which emerge co-created, negotiated and transient meanings. In contemporary performance practice, the intersubjective space reflects ways in which performer and audience in their interdependent subjectivities create shared meaning through a process of co-authorship (Radosavljević, 2013). This is most exemplified in practices such as relational performances (O'Grady, 2013) that place the spectator as co-creator of the performance event whose shape and meaning becomes the expression of an intersubjective encounter. In such practices, the participants determine the course of the performance as well as being determined by it by virtue of partaking in a communal process (Fischer-Lichte, 2008). The theatre artist Adrian Howells exemplifies such practice in the context of autobiographical work whereby artist and spectator mutually define and shape the performance through the quality of their intimate encounter in the moment (Heddon & Howells, 2011).

A Conceptual Framework for Autobiographical Performance: The Five Witnesses

My discussion so far has positioned AP within a web of interactions and influences reflecting various degrees of tension within this art and therapeutic form. This brings me to suggest a relational model that conceptualizes the way in which the production of meaning within the autobiographical space results from constant negotiations and transactions with multi-layered contexts that I will refer to as *witnesses*. I have identified five layers of witnessing and I have centered this model on the performance object as being an expression of these transactions but also enabling renewed ways of relating to oneself and others.

The *internal witness* refers to the performer becoming a witness to himself/herself (Jones, 2007), and to the self entering a dialogue with the self (Heddon, 2013). But as one of the characters in Pirandello's *Six Characters in Search of An Author* says: 'This is the real drama for me; the belief that we all think of ourselves as one single person: but it's not true: each of us is several different people, and all these people live inside us' (1988, p. 92). Heddon (2013) compares AP to a hall of mirrors whereby different selves coexist (Hermans, Kempen, & Van Loon, 1992) and enter in a dialogue with one another resulting in new awareness and understanding.

The *engaged witness* refers to the members of a group working together on APs, being a witnessing audience (Rubin, 2007), and sometimes physically engaged with each other's work. This is particularly exemplified in student trainings and with client groups. The witnessing emerges from the concurrent positions of being witness to others and being witnessed by others (Jones, 2005). The nature of the group matrix and of the interactions within it will have a particular bearing on the way individuals approach their performance. Equally, the way in which the different performed narratives will be experienced in the group will in turn generate new narratives and define the contours of their intertextual meaning.

The *active witness* (Jones, 1993) refers to the person of the dramatherapist, whose presence constitutes a unique and singular factor in the devising and performing of autobiographical material. The dramatherapist acts as container of the experiences, emotions and interactions occurring within a group. S/he holds the boundaries of the space and safeguards the well-being of those involved. S/he plays a range of roles (facilitator, mediator, director) that involve various levels of engagement and that could be equally conducive to creativity or tension. Moreover, s/he will be subject to transference and countertransference in relationships. S/he will evoke feelings in those in the group and s/he will find herself/himself exposed to experiences that may connect to her/his own autobiographical memory.

The *observing witness* refers to the external audience coming to see a performance. The audience bears witness to a performed experience with possible profound healing effects on the performer. Its level of engagement will vary depending on the aesthetic choices made by the performer and on the intentions to reach out. Nonetheless, the audience largely remains an unknown entity whose reaction and position vis-à-vis the performance cannot be fully predicted. Is it justified to see the audience as an undifferentiated entity of individuals? If this audience is often experienced as supportive and empathetic, wouldn't it be presumptuous to believe that it is invariably benevolent? Different audiences, whether or not preselected, will experience and will be experienced differently with significant effects on the way the performer will present on stage.

The *silent witness* refers to the larger historical and cultural context that permeates individual histories leaving social imprints on the way experience is assimilated and communicated. It is the equivalent to what Hopper calls the *social unconscious* (Hopper & Weinberg, 2011), or a set of social, political, cultural and discursive structures and practices that define the domains of the possible and are sedimented, would say Butler (1997), within the body and the psyche. This is where the performance object becomes the expression of the interplay and tension between the private and the public, between constraint and freedom.

METHODOLOGICAL IMPLICATIONS

I have attempted in this chapter to offer a theoretical discussion on how the production of meaning in AP can be described as emerging from different layers of intersubjective relationships within the performance space, as suggested above in the conceptual framework of the five witnesses. I will conclude with some brief remarks on the methodological implications for research of this epistemological framework.

First, it seems important to identify a methodology that takes as unit of analysis the different *levels of intersubjectivity* within the relational framework. These different levels are the interactions between group members including the therapist, the intertextual relationships between performed narratives in their form and content, the relationship of the individual group members with themselves, and the relationship to an external audience.

Second, performance as an embodied practice requires an embodied methodology (Pelias, 2008) that investigates the way in which the body is a receptacle of tension and intersubjective dynamics, and how these get experienced and communicated in a performance context.

Finally, intersubjectivity suggests dialogue as an epistemological and methodological vehicle. It points towards the creation of a community of inquiry between researcher and participants based on a dialogic collaborative process (Paulus, Woodside, & Ziegler, 2008), whereby the different voices of researcher and participants are in a constant and iterative dialogue on the nature of the meaning of their mutual experiences. It suggests a methodology that would elucidate the way in which the production of meaning in AP can be described as resulting from a contextualized and situated intersubjective co-creation. This chapter has proposed how such a co-creation is the expression of relational processes and interactions between different levels of witnessing in autobiographical performance in dramatherapy.

REFERENCES

Bakhtin, M. (1986). *Speech genres & other late essays.* Austin: University of Texas Press.

Bakhtin, M. (1990). *Art and answerability.* Austin: University of Texas Press.

Barthes, R. (1977). *Image, music, text.* London: Fontana Press.

Benjamin, J. (1995). *Like subjects, love objects: Essays on recognition and sexual difference.* New Haven: Yale University Press.

Benjamin, W. (1999). The storyteller. In W. Benjamin (Ed.), *Illuminations* (pp. 83–107). London: Pimlico.

Benjamin, J. (2004). Beyond doer and done to: An intersubjective view of thirdness. *Psychoanalytic Quarterly, 73,* 5–46.

Bennett, S. (1997). *Theatre audiences: A theory of production and reception.* London: Routledge.

Boenisch, P. M. (2010). Towards a theatre of encounter and experience: Reflexive dramaturgies and classic texts. *Contemporary Theatre Review, 20*(2), 162–172.

Brook, P. (1990). *The empty space*. London: Penguin Books.

Bruner, J. (1986). *Actual minds, possible worlds*. Cambridge: Harvard University Press.

Butler, J. (1993). Critically queer. *GlQ: A Journal of Gay and Lesbian Studies, 1*, 17–32.

Butler, J. (1997). *Excitable speech: A politics of the performative*. London: Routledge.

Calle, S. (2003). *Douleur exquise*. Arles: Actes Sud.

Conquerwood, D. (1985). Performing as a moral act: Ethical dimensions of the ethnography of performance. *Literature in Performance, 5*(2), 1–13.

Cornejo, C. (2008). Intersubjectivity as co-phenomenology. *Integrative Psychology of Behavior, 42*, 171–178.

Czarniawska, B. (2004). *Narratives in social science research*. London: Sage Publications.

Emunah, R. (1994). *Acting for real*. New York: Brunner-Mazel.

Emunah, R. (2015). Self-revelatory performance: A form of drama therapy and theatre. *Drama Therapy Review, 1*(1), 71–85.

Fischer-Lichte, E. (2008). *The transformative power of performance*. Abingdon: Routledge.

Fitzpatrick, L. (2011). The performance of violence and the ethics of spectatorship. *Performance Research, 16*(1), 59–67.

Grainger, R. (2005). Theatre and encounter Part III—Transforming theatre. *Dramatherapy, 27*(1), 8–12.

Grotowski, J. (1991). *Towards a poor theatre*. London: Methuen Drama.

Heddon, D. (2008). *Autobiography and performance*. New York: Palgrave MacMillan.

Heddon, D. (2013). Beyond the self: Autobiography as dialogue. In C. Wallace (Ed.), *Monologues: Theatre, performance, subjectivity* (pp. 157–184). Prague: Litteraria Pragensia.

Heddon, D., & Howells, A. (2011). From talking to silence: A confessional journey. *PAJ: Journal of Performance and Art, 33*(1), 1–12.

Hermans, H., Kempen, H., & Van Loon, R. (1992). The dialogical self: Beyond individualism and rationalism. *American Psychologist, 47*(1), 23–33.

Holland, D., Lachicotte, W., Skinner, D., & Cain, C. (2001). *Identity and agency in cultural worlds*. Cambridge: Harvard University Press.

Hopper, K., & Weinberg, H. (Eds.). (2011). *The social unconscious in persons, groups and societies*. London: Karnac.

Jones, P. (1993). The active witness: The acquisition of meaning in dramatherapy. In H. Payne (Ed.), *Handbook of inquiry in the arts therapies: One river, many currents* (pp. 41–55). London: Jessica Kingsley Publishers.

Jones, P. (2005). *The arts therapies: A revolution in healthcare*. Hove: Brunner-Routledge.

Jones, P. (2007). *Drama as therapy: Theory, practice and research*. London: Routledge.

Levinas, E. (1989). *The Levinas reader*. Oxford: Blackwell.

MacKay, B. (1996). Brief dramatherapy and the collective creation. In A. Gersie (Ed.), *Dramatic approaches to brief therapy* (pp. 161–174). London: Jessica Kingsley.

Madison, D. S. (2007). Co-performative witnessing. *Cultural Studies, 21*(6), 826–831.

Marranca, B. (1979). The self as text: Uses of autobiography in the theatre. *Performing Arts Journal, 4*(1/2), 85–105.

McAdams, D. P., & McLean, K. C. (2013). Narrative identity. *Current Directions in Psychological Science, 22*, 233–238.

McAdams, D. P., Josselson, R., & Lieblich, A. (2006). *Identity and story: Creating self in narrative*. Washington: American Psychological Association.

McLean, K. C., Pasupathi, M., & Pals, J. L. (2007). Selves creating stories creating selves: A process model of self-development. *Personality and Social Psychology Review, 11*, 262–278.

Merleau-Ponty, M. (1962). *Phenomenology of perception*. London: Routledge.

Nolan, P. (2012). *Therapist and client: A relational approach to psychotherapy*. Chichester: Wiley-Blackwell.

O'Grady, A. (2013). Exploring radical openness: A porous model for relational festival performance. *Studies in Theatre and Performance, 33*(2), 133–151.

Paulus, T., Woodside, M., & Ziegler, M. (2008). Extending the conversation: Qualitative research as dialogic collaborative process. *The Qualitative Report, 13*(2), 226–243.

Payne, M. (2006). *Narrative therapy*. London: Sage Publications.

Pelias, R. J. (2008). Performative inquiry: Embodiment and its challenges. In J. G. Knowles & A. L. Cole (Eds.), *Handbook of the Arts in Qualitative Research* (pp. 185–193). London: Sage Publications.

Phelan, P. (2004). Marina Abramović: Witnessing shadows. *Theatre Journal, 56*(4), 569–577.

Pirandello, L. (1988). *Three plays*. London: Methuen Drama.

Pitches, J. (2003). *Vsevolod Meyerhold*. London: Routledge.

Pitruzzella, S. (2009). The audience role in theatre and dramatherapy. *Dramatherapy, 31*(1), 10–14.

Radosavljević, D. (2013). *Theatre-making: Interplay between text and performance in the 21st century*. Basingstoke: Palgrave Macmillan.

Rancière, J. (2011). *The emancipated spectator*. London: Verso.

Rosenblatt, L. M. (1994). *The reader, the text, the poem: The transactional theory of the literary work*. Carbondale and Edwardsville: Southern Illinois University Press.

Rozik, E. (2010). *Generating theatre meaning*. Brighton: Sussex Academic Press.

Rubin, S. (2007). Self-revelatory performance. In A. Blatner (Ed.), *Interactive and improvisational drama: Varieties of applied theatre and performance* (pp. 250–259). Lincoln: iUniverse.

Sajnani, N. (2012). The implicated witness: Towards a relational aesthetic in dramatherapy. *Dramatherapy, 34*(1), 6–21.

Schrader, C. (1998). The studio upstairs: Performance as a way of relating to the world. *Dramatherapy, 20*(2), 15–19.

Shepherd, S., & Wallis, M. (2004). *Drama/theatre/performance*. London: Routledge.

Smagorinski, P. (2001). If meaning is constructed, what's it made from? *Review of Educational Research, 71*(1), 133–169.

Stern, R. (2002). *Hegel and the phenomenology of spirit*. Abingdon: Routledge.

Todorov, T. (1984). *Mikhail Bakhtin: The dialogical principle*. Minneapolis: University of Minnesota Press.

Wood, S. (2015). Performing stories of lived experience. *Dramascope*. Accessed January 27, 2015, from https://thedramascope.wordpress.com/2015/01/27/performing-stories-of-lived-experience/

PART II

Applications and Approaches

CHAPTER 8

Autobiographical Therapeutic Performance as Individual Therapy

Armand Volkas

These are some of the themes and plots of *autobiographical therapeutic performances* (ATP) that I have assisted my clients in giving birth to and directed. At the end of a performance, when the actor has bared her soul through the enactment of her story, she stands psychically naked onstage in a trance before her witnesses. She bows humbly, defiantly, triumphantly, dissociated, or with quiet disbelief that she has actually reached this moment of completion. The spell is broken by the audience's applause, the standing ovation or the stunned silence of profound empathy for the performer and the courageous emotional risks that she took to reveal herself before those gathered to support her.

A woman reclaims her power and self-love in the face of an absent father, 'taming the wolf' within her that threatens to devour her self-esteem.
A man born into enormous wealth makes peace with his privilege and a larger than life father.
A French woman uncovers a family secret about an ancestor—a Catholic priest who fathered a child with an African slave in Argentina. She moves into a deep exploration of the metaphor of enslavement by men and unshackles herself from the oppression of patriarchy.

A. Volkas, MA, MFA, MFT, RDT-BCT (✉)
California Institute of Integral Studies, San Francisco, CA, USA

Living Arts Counseling Center, Emeryville, CA, USA
e-mail: armandvolkas@gmail.com

© The Author(s) 2016
S. Pendzik et al. (eds.), *The Self in Performance*,
DOI 10.1057/978-1-137-53593-1_8

Months before the performance, at the beginning of the creation process, clients who choose to engage in an ATP meet with their director/
therapist and decide on an intention, a therapeutic goal, a trauma, a mission, an image or an issue that they want to delve into. A therapeutic contract emerges over time. Through improvisational exploration, dreaming,
journaling, writing scenes and monologues, the director/therapist guides
the client towards the momentous performance date.

On this pivotal day, clients know that they may be changed forever. As
in a *hero's journey* (Campbell, 1972), performers go on a quest to heal
themselves, fighting their inner demons and dragons, and entering into a
no-man's land where they are betwixt and between (Turner, 1967). This
is the liminal state, the stripping away of what one has been, but not yet
arrived at whom one will become. In many ways, the ATP is an initiation
rite, a rite of passage marking entrance or acceptance into a group or society (Van Gennep, 1960). In a wider psychological sense, the performance
signifies a transformation in which the initiate is reborn into a new role.

The process of psychotherapy itself often follows an initiation rite structure—embarking on a journey towards change, confronting the unknown
and returning to a changed self. What is different in ATP is that the spiritual and emotional emergency, often necessary for therapeutic change to
occur, is self-induced by the client, with the guidance of the therapist/
director. This complex, heightened internal drama takes place under the
pressure of the impending performance. Go forward, embrace the change,
or face the humiliation of failure in front of the tribal witnesses gathered
to attest to your courage. In ATP, the looming performance date creates
the feeling of urgency essential for the client to completely commit to the
creation process. The issues being worked on are elevated to a crisis that
calls for transformation.

In the post-performance dénouement, the guests often stand in a
queue, resembling a wedding receiving line, taking turns to share their
congratulations and the impact the ATP has had on them. A wedding is an
apt metaphor for this event. However, the actor is not marrying another
person, but symbolically marrying herself.

Since the 1980s, when I first began performing and directing autobiographical performances, I have seen this rite of passage ritual play itself
out in this manner hundreds of times. From ten-minute scenes as the
culmination of a course on drama therapy to the graduation ritual that it
has become for many drama therapy programs throughout the world, to
hour-long theatre pieces created in the context of a private practice and

performed for the public, I have witnessed the transformative effects of this form. In this chapter, I review my method of accompanying clients in individual therapy through this process, using the main theoretical frameworks that inform my practice of ATP: the hero's journey, the rite of passage, and *Transactional Analysis*.

THE HERO'S JOURNEY

The archetypal image of the hero's journey, found in stories and myths, is widely recognized around the world. It has a useful prototypical story structure that may also serve as a powerful metaphor for the ATP journey, and has been outlined by mythologist, Joseph Campbell (1972) as follows: An adventurer hears a call to discovery and separates from the everyday world, setting out on a journey filled with dangers. The hero experiences many difficult challenges and tests, each rich with learning. Ultimately, the hero confronts a seemingly insurmountable challenge—a supreme test that cannot be overcome with physical capacities alone. To be successful, the hero must reach beyond his ego into a spiritual realm in which he awakens to a new and more soulful relationship with himself, with other people, and with the universe. With this spiritual initiation, the hero then makes a journey of return, bringing these gifts of insight back to the larger community.

The ATP process often taps into the archetypal pattern of the classic hero's journey: The client embarks on a journey of self-discovery and change, is tested by internal or external forces and, almost always, returns triumphant. This therapeutic narrative perhaps helps to explain why the return from an ATP process often holds so much meaning and power for those embarking on it, as the journey entails a metaphorical voyage into intra-psychic levels, along with artistic disclosure in front of an audience.

My own calling for working in this way comes out of my own personal journey: In 1975, in response to my historical inheritance as a child of resistance fighters and survivors of Auschwitz, I brought together a group of children of Holocaust survivors in their 20s to create a theatre piece on the legacy of the Holocaust (Volkas, 2009). This was at a time when Holocaust survivors were just beginning to reveal their traumatic experiences to the wider world. At the same time, these survivors' descendants were discovering the ways in which their experiences paralleled each other (Epstein, 1979). Exploring the transgenerational nature of the trauma, *Survivors* premiered in Los Angeles in 1976. It had a long run followed by an extensive college tour. This autobiographical theatre piece arose from the personal lives and research of the actors, with me functioning as director, editor and dramaturge.

In 1987, I created a solo full-length ATP after being hired by a public defender as a drama therapist to work with a defendant before his high-profile death penalty trial. He had been convicted of murdering a man, woman and an 18-month-old child, with a knife. For over one year before his trial and conviction, I had repeated drama therapy sessions with this man in a holding cell, which was continually patrolled by prison guards. These encounters ultimately stirred up complex feelings within me. Working with him triggered my countertransference as the son of Holocaust survivors and provoked deep investigations of the role of perpetrator and my own capacity for extreme cruelty. I also struggled with an ethical question. Was it ethical to use the tools of drama therapy to aid a murderer? If the defendant had been a Mafioso instead of a very emotionally wounded young man, could I have still taken on this case? Interviewed by the press after the trial, the jury revealed that my humanizing testimony during the penalty phase apparently contributed to the defendant receiving life imprisonment, instead of death by lethal injection. In the aftermath of this experience, filled with difficult emotions and intense existential and spiritual questions, I felt the need to explore my own feelings further by shaping them into an ATP, a process that allowed me to heal myself and continue with my research in understanding the impact of direct and inherited trauma. *The Murderer Within* was first performed at the NADT Conference in Los Angeles in 1988 with my drama therapy colleagues as witnesses.

ATP as a Rite of Passage

A rite of passage is a transition ritual that helps an individual to move from one social state to another—from adolescence to adulthood, from student to graduate, from apprentice to full member of a profession, from being single to being married. It transforms both the society's definition of the individual and the individual's self-perception. Such rituals of social transition mark socially recognized stages of life and help the individual and the group to adjust to the new status and its implications for behavior and social relations (Turner 1969; Van Gennep, 1960).

Though not a socially recognized rite of passage, ATP processes can provide a path through which therapeutic change can occur. With the breakdown in modern societies of meaningful rituals that help people through life transitions, ATP offers a drama-therapeutic structure for clients to move from one state of being to another—from grief and loss to embracing life again, from rage at an absent parent to making peace with the limitations of the parent that they had, from a state of fear to finding courage and standing up for their own emotional rights.

According to Van Gennep (1960) and Turner (1969), rites of passage generally involve three principal phases:

1. Separating the individuals involved from their preceding social state.
2. A period of transition or initiation in which they are neither one thing nor the other.
3. A reintegration phase during which, through various rites of incorporation, they are absorbed into their new social state.

The most prominent feature of all rites of passage is its transitional nature. Rites of passage always involve what Victor Turner (1969) has called *liminality*, the stage of being neither here nor there—no longer part of the old and not yet part of the new. One of the chief characteristics of this liminal period in any rite of passage is the gradual psychological opening of the initiates to their profound interior changes. In many initiation rites involving major transitions into new social roles, this openness is achieved through rituals designed to break down the initiate's belief system—the internal mental structures of concepts and categories through which they perceive and interpret the world and their relationship to it (Floyd, 2003).

Similar feelings of psychological opening up and the breakdown of old belief systems are reported by many ATP clients, as they describe their experience of personal transformation.

ATP AS A FORM OF INDIVIDUAL DRAMA THERAPY

Renée Emunah has applied therapeutic theatre with elements of what she later called *self-revelatory performance* (Self-Rev) with psychiatric and ex-psychiatric patients since 1979 (Emunah, 1994; Emunah & Johnson, 1983). In the last two decades, the Self-Rev model continued to expand primarily as a culmination of students' training in drama therapy (Rubin, 2007; Emunah, Raucher & Ramirez, 2014). Emunah (2015) has articulated Self-Rev as a form of theatre and drama therapy, with a strong emphasis on aesthetic quality, and therefore most suitable for people who are already trained actors and/or drama therapists. Yet my view of the form has evolved in a different direction, as I have been using ATP in the context of private practice as a psychotherapist and as the Clinical Director of The Living Arts Counseling Center. In these contexts, aesthetics and acting skills are acquired as part of the therapeutic process. In addition, the setting for the work (including production-related issues, payment for hours extending beyond the usual psychotherapy meetings, etc.) are negotiated and addressed as therapeutic material, and the witnesses of the performance are carefully chosen by the clients, as part of the therapeutic process.

In a field as young as drama therapy, terminology of various approaches are still evolving as evidenced by the multiple names used by the authors in this book to describe their work. While I have been informed and influenced by the powerful form of self-revelatory performance that Renée Emunah (1994) was the first to articulate, the term Self-Rev has always felt incomplete to me as a description of what I do. Being directly involved in presenting the approach to the public and in acquainting potential clients with the transformative power of drama therapy, I find the word 'therapeutic' a crucial one to communicate what is at the heart of this form.

I believe that ATP is not just a form for drama therapy students and actors, but has great potential as a form of individual drama therapy for any client seeking personal growth and change, who has enough ego strength to withstand the intensity of and commitment to such a journey. Here are three examples of contexts in which I have used ATP. My focus in the rest of this chapter will be on the third type:

1. Cyclical performances by members of an ongoing drama therapy group. For example, on three occasions a year each participant creates a theatre piece reflecting their current issue and invites safe audience members to witness their growth.
2. A time-limited group specifically organized to support each member's creation and performance of their own ATP, which I call *Acts of Witness*. Developed in collaboration with psychotherapist and drama therapist Jennifer Stuckert, Acts of Witness combines the weekly support of a community of clients all on the same creative journey. I co-lead the weekly group explorations and the clients receive the additional attention of a designated drama therapist/director who guides the ATP actor/client in weekly rehearsals leading to a public performance.

3. ATP performances created in the context of individual therapy. Weekly sessions ultimately lead to a performance in a theatre, which brings a therapeutic process to a new stage. A typical ATP process can range from three to five months; weekly sessions start at 1.5 hours and increase in length and intensity as the performance date draws nearer.

ATP in the Context of Transactional Analysis

Having been trained in Transactional Analysis, some of the core concepts of this form of psychotherapy have influenced my approach to ATP. Transactional Analysis (TA) is based on the premise that each human being has three observable ego states or roles: parent, adult and child. The goal in TA is to ensure clients regain autonomy over their lives. The creator of TA, Eric Berne (1961), defined this process as the recovery of three vital human capacities—spontaneity, awareness and intimacy. TA is a widely recognized form of psychotherapy that involves a set of tools designed to promote personal growth and change. Tools from TA that have a bearing on ATP include therapeutic contracts, life scripts and re-decision.

Therapeutic Contracts

One of the most important aspects of my approach to ATP is the idea of the therapeutic contract. Borrowed from TA, the contract is a mutual agreement entered into by client and therapist to pursue specific changes that the client desires. The contract contains statements of objectives that the client will attain and the criteria to determine when these goals have been effectively met.

When applied to ATP, the contract is flexible and can be refined as we proceed. The first iteration of the contract can be simply to experiment with images and improvisations in order to reveal what clients want or need to change in their lives. Refining and clarifying the contract is an ongoing process. Within the first phases of the exploration, clients may work through several possible ideas for what their piece is going to be about. The therapist/director continually redirects them to focus on the statements they want to make to their witnesses. This contract becomes the compass that guides clients on their journey.

A good example of a therapeutic contract in ATP is one that was entered into with a client of German descent who wanted to explore her blocks to intimacy. She had been in a series of failed relationships and committed to unearthing her unconscious patterns that could be affecting the way she relates to men. The guiding question in our explorations became, 'what is preventing her from opening up her heart and getting close?'

Ultimately, her improvisational investigations led to the image of a chest of secrets being ferociously guarded by a paranoid alter-ego. This character emerged from a suggestion I made about using the box as a metaphor for her closing off her emotions and vulnerability and was loosely based on her psychotic aunt who had inherited the belongings of her Nazi father after World War II. Her aunt kept her father's medals from Hitler, as well as other documents, hidden in a box. In the unfolding of the ATP piece, this alter-ego slowly reveals her grandfather's imagined acts of perpetration. Also revealed are her mother's wounding and abandonment by her father, who was removed from the family after the war, and the client's own role as a parentified child caretaker. As we delved into the client's relationship history and childhood wounding in action, as well as historical trauma, it became clear to me that the theatre piece could be about several of the themes that appeared through her improvisational explorations: a specific man who had broken her heart; her mother's confusing messages about love; or owning her power and sensuality as a woman.

These were all compelling issues to address. However, under the time pressure of a scheduled performance date, I reminded my client that although she wanted to put everything into her piece, she needed to choose the images and scenes that most powerfully depicted her struggle with intimacy. One of my roles as her drama therapist/director was to use the therapeutic contract to help keep her focused on her goal. The contract then became the litmus test for what images or scenes stayed in the piece and which ones ended up on the cutting room floor.

Towards the end of her performance she speaks to an imaginary future lover, '*Here I am in all my naked ugliness. Can you love me? Do you see me? Can you love all of this?*'

The client's defenses stripped away in front of the audience, her vulnerability and desire to be seen powerfully revealed and her deep yearning to be loved unconditionally displayed, it was clear that she had taken a courageous step towards opening her heart to the possibility of loving again. I believe that this could be traced back to the central guiding therapeutic contract at the beginning of the process.

Coming up with the initial contract is akin to the hero embarking on the journey. Clients set out on their creative and therapeutic quests with a sense of direction as they travel into uncharted emotional territory. The stating, restating, and the ongoing clarification and refining of the therapeutic objectives represent the series of challenges the hero faces along the way.

Uncovering Unconscious Life Scripts

Transactional Analysis proposes that dysfunctional behavior is the result of self-limiting decisions made in childhood, in the interest of survival. Such decisions culminate in what Berne (1961) and Steiner (1974) called the *life script*—the unconscious life plan that governs the way life is lived out. Uncovering and changing the life script is one of the central aims of TA psychotherapy.

Through drama therapy, theatre transformations and psychodramatic exercises, spoken and unspoken parental and societal messages and injunctions such as 'Don't be separate from me,' 'Don't grow up,' 'Don't need,' 'Don't trust,' or 'Don't get close' are uncovered. These injunctions reveal the dysfunctional life script that the client is living.

One client, who I will call Victoria, provides a good example of the unveiling of a sabotaging life script and the creation of a new hopeful narrative. She created and performed two separate, but related solo ATP pieces over a period of ten months. A summary of her transformative process follows:

Raised by a mother who had absorbed and transmitted the misogynistic messages towards women in her society, Victoria, a South American immigrant, sought therapy for her depression. After a childhood characterized by emotional neglect and physical abuse by her mother and abandonment by her father, Victoria tried to escape her fate and her suicidal life script. 'Don't be powerful,' 'Don't be successful,' 'Don't think,' 'Don't need,' 'Don't be,' were among the debilitating messages that she received from her family. At the same time, however, Victoria also held enormous strength and resilience in the face of her life's circumstances.

Victoria entered into a therapeutic contract to grieve her deep losses, and transform her life script filled with victimization into an empowered and life-affirming narrative. In her first ATP, Victoria revealed her story of abuse and neglect through monologues and scenes: Throughout the piece, she is pursued by a vicious and punishing inner tormentor—a force that takes the form of a Swordsman. Running in place to symbolize her flight from hopelessness, she tries to escape her reality:

I'm not going back, I won't go back. I'm leaving this prison.

In a metaphorical dance, Victoria misguidedly tries to escape and find solace in drugs, alcohol and sex, but the Swordsman finally catches up with her. In a venomous and vicious rant, the Swordsman (also played by Victoria) attacks her competence, her attempts to better herself, her sadness and her aging:

'You'll end up old, poor, powerless and alone. What's the point!' he concludes.

On all fours, Victoria exposes her neck to the Swordsman:

'Go ahead, do it! CUT IT OFF! CUT IT OFF!' she says to him.

In slow motion, the Swordsman cuts off her head. Victoria falls to the floor and, in a transition, moves deeply into her grief:

I mourn for the family I never had
I grieve for the cruelty inflicted upon me
I mourn for all my hopes and dreams that never came true

As Victoria stops crying, the scene transforms into a dream world. She sees a mountain and climbs to the top. Before her, she sees a chasm and walks closer to the edge and looks down.

I see a bottomless chasm. Below, I see my annihilation.

She looks across the abyss. On the other side she sees a Beckoner. The Beckoner, also played by Victoria, extends her hand and calls for her. She implores Victoria to jump across:

Don't look down at the chasm. Just jump! Come on! I'll catch you!

Victoria hesitates. She demands a guarantee from the Beckoner who responds:

No guarantees, but yes, on this side you have the power to do everything you possibly can to choose and create meaning in your life. Come on! Jump! I'll catch you!

Victoria takes a moment to consider her choices. She slowly takes a step back and, running in slow motion, leaps across the chasm. But the lights fade out before the audience knows whether she made it to the other side or not.

Although not actively suicidal, Victoria's deep hopelessness and tragic life script were exposed by the ATP process. Having lived her life trying to escape her difficult circumstances and battling her brutal inner critic, she viewed her life as being a failure. Victoria faced a decision in both her life and in the script she was writing. As the performance drew near, we struggled to find an ending to the piece in rehearsals. Her drama refused to be wrapped up neatly in a nice bow. As her therapist/director, I proposed the metaphor of approaching two cliffs separated by a chasm; we spent several sessions working psychodramatically and metaphorically, standing at the precipice facing the Beckoner, who represented her fragile hope for a meaningful life. Victoria could not decide whether she would take the perilous jump and was not yet ready to find out. I, as therapist, felt torn between challenging her and respecting her process; both of us seemed caught in liminal space. Leaving Victoria in the middle of a crisis on the existential stage was the authentic place to end the piece. She felt at peace with this decision. The outcome would need to be decided in a future ATP. When she performed this piece for an invited audience, their response to this uncertain ending was a stunned awe.

Transforming the Life Script

A few months later, after several post-performance follow-up therapy sessions, Victoria decided she wanted to do a second ATP, which would begin at the moment where the last piece ended. In sessions, Victoria explored the images, metaphors and themes that bubbled up from the depths of her unconscious, including the historical trauma of the subjugation of her ancestors, the South American indigenous people that live within her, as well as her identity as a *mestiza*.

Her second ATP began with her jump across the abyss. This time she makes it to the other side. However, Victoria finds herself in a jungle and the Beckoner is nowhere to be found. She had taken the risk to hope and now feels betrayed. The *law of the jungle* becomes a metaphor for her precarious life. She finds herself in a dream-like world, full of Amazonian cannibals, panthers, and Spanish conquistadors, left to make her way on her own without support. She hunts and forages and learns how to survive in the jungle, becoming one with nature. She finds a mate. One day, Victoria is shot by both a gun and an arrow and faints. She wakes up to find herself being nurtured by the Beckoner who has transformed into the role of a Nurturer. As the woman stirs an imaginary cauldron of soup, she adds pinches of spices to the nourishing mixture describing their properties, such as:

> *Determination: to overcome your demons so you can stay engaged in the living of life.*
> *Love: to be able to love yourself so you can accept and celebrate your strengths and have empathy for your weaknesses.*
> *Compassion: to keep your heart open in the face of hate and rage.*

After adding other strengths to the soup, the Nurturer begins to feed Victoria saying,

> *You've been through a lot. All the pain and isolation, all the anguish and deep loneliness, but I'm here for you now and I love you and I will continue to love you until the day you die.*

Then the Nurturer brings Victoria's attention to the witnesses in the audience, saying:

> *Look at all these wonderful people who came to support you. Some of them know you well and some are only beginning to know you, but they're all here to support you. So go ahead, you can feel proud of the courage it took to reach in and reach out and expose yourself this way—go ahead take your bow. I'll be standing right here next to you.*
> *Victoria bows to the audience.*

The brutal Swordsman of her previous ATP was replaced by the Beckoner, a nurturing and protective parental figure who had begun to grow inside of Victoria. In TA, the idea of re-parenting yourself is a central concept and part of transforming one's life script (James, 1981). Inviting trustworthy friends to witness and support transformation creates external emotional resourcing along with the internal resourcing of self re-parenting.

The Role of the Reparative Witness

In many contexts in which ATPs are presented, the performances are open to the general public. The performer/client has no control over who will witness her deeply personal piece. Some verbal guidelines are given to audience members about how to approach the performers after their presentation, as they are often in a vulnerable state. My approach to ATP includes the distinct role of what I call the *reparative witness*. In ATP, witnessing should not be a passive act, but an integral component of the therapeutic process. Witnessing provides a reparative holding and mirroring experience for the client. In the context of individual psychotherapy work, it is particularly important that clients be able to invite their witnesses based on trust: they constitute the client's support system, which will ultimately function as the healing family and help the client maintain the therapeutic change. As performing an ATP can be such a public act that often leaves clients in an exposed and altered state, I believe care needs to be taken in helping the ATP client bridge the therapeutic process with the worlds to which they are returning.

RE-DECISION

This term refers to an individual's capacity to re-decide and alter certain decisions made as a child, which stem from unconscious scripts (Goulding & Goulding, 1979). Re-decision reflects the assumption in TA therapy that individuals have the potential to lead their lives as they choose.

In my approach to ATP, the hero's journey is, in essence, a journey of re-decision. Most ATPs that I have seen follow this structure. For example, a client goes on a quest to rescue their inner child; they fight their inner demons in some form, and then become the hero of their own story. They decide to prevail. Here is an example of a moment of re-decision in an ATP I directed:

In the throes of hopelessness, the grandson of Auschwitz survivors asks God,

> *Why does my mother hate me so much? What have I done to deserve this? I must have done something terrible. I see the hate in her eyes. She despises me. I am the reason for all of her unhappiness. I'm damaged beyond repair. She wants me to disappear. I must erase myself. I must kill the resilient spirit within me that she despises so much.*

In a theatrical physicalization of his struggle with his impulse to annihilate himself, the moment of re-decision and transformation occurs:

> *Enough! Stop! I must stop the abuse. I will not transmit this abuse. The abuse must stop here! The abuse stops here.*

Before his gathered witnesses, he goes on to reclaim his emotional rights, violated by the domino effect of historical trauma.

I have the right to breathe. I have the right to take up space in the world. I have the right to feel—to be part of humanity. I have the right to walk through this world without self-hate. I have the right to be wanted. To be loved. I have a right to my curiosity. I have a right to have a body and for this body not to be violated, I have a right to set boundaries and to protect myself. I have a right to need and have needs. I have a right to live without fear of annihilation...I have the right to exist!

The actor then transforms into an American soldier who liberates the child from Auschwitz, adopts him and promises to re-parent him.

CONCLUSION

Autobiographical therapeutic performance provides clients seeking personal growth and change the opportunity to give aesthetic form to the wounding experiences and negative messages that have shaped them. It can transform and reintegrate their traumas into a new life-affirming sense of self and an emotionally generative life script. ATP organically follows a rite of passage and hero's journey structure, which can be useful metaphors in guiding both the development of the theatre piece and the therapeutic process. Furthermore, Transactional Analysis concepts can be used as a therapeutic template, integrating and adapting ideas such as the therapeutic contract, life script and re-decision to the ATP process, as well as adding a special emphasis on the role of reparative witness.

Because the ATP process aligns with the timelessness of the archetypal hero's journey, it gets to the source of the actor's primal wounding and fuels the fires of their creativity. It taps into the actor's desire to be seen and elevates their story to mythic proportions. It paints their individual struggles with a collective brush, connecting to the existential and universal dilemmas we all face.

REFERENCES

Berne, E. (1961). *Transactional analysis in psychotherapy: A systematic individual and social psychiatry.* New York: Grove Press.
Campbell, J. (1972). *The hero with a thousand faces* (2nd ed.). Princeton, NJ: Princeton University Press.

Emunah, R. (1994). *Acting for real: Drama therapy process, technique, and performance*. New York: Brunner-Mazel.

Emunah, R. (2015). Self-revelatory performance: A form of drama therapy and theatre. *Drama Therapy Review, 1*(1), 71–85.

Emunah, R., & Johnson, D. R. (1983). The impact of theatrical performance on the self images of psychiatric patients. *Arts in Psychotherapy, 10*, 233–239.

Emunah, R., Raucher, G., & Ramirez, A. (2014). Self-revelatory performance in mitigating the impact of trauma. In N. Sajnani & D. Johnson (Eds.), *Trauma informed drama therapy* (pp. 93–121). Springfield, IL: Charles Thomas.

Epstein, H. (1979). *Children of the Holocaust: Conversations with sons and daughters of survivors*. New York: Putnam.

Floyd, R. (2003). *Birth as an American rite of passage* (2nd ed.). Berkeley, CA: University of California Press.

Goulding, M., & Goulding, R. (1979). *Changing lives through redecision therapy*. New York: Brunner-Mazel.

James, M. (1981). *Breaking free: Self-reparenting for a new life*. Reading, MA: Addison-Wesley.

Rubin, S. (2007). Self-revelatory performance. In A. Blatner (Ed.), *Interactive and improvisational drama: Varieties of applied theatre and performance* (pp. 250–259). New York: iUniverse.

Steiner, C. (1974). *Scripts people live: Transactional analysis of life scripts*. New York: Grove Press.

Turner, V. (1967). *The forest of symbols: Aspects of Ndembu ritual*. Ithaca, NY: Cornell University Press.

Turner, V. (1969). *The ritual process: Structure and anti-structure*. Chicago: Aldine Publishers.

Van Gennep, A. (1960). *The rites of passage*. Chicago, IL: University of Chicago Press.

Volkas, A. (2009). Healing the wounds of history: Drama therapy in collective trauma and intercultural conflict resolution. In D. Johnson & R. Emunah (Eds.), *Current approaches in drama therapy* (pp. 145–171). Springfield, IL: Charles C. Thomas.

CHAPTER 9

Embodied Life Stories: Transforming Shame Through Self-Revelatory Performance

Sheila Rubin

The experience of seeing oneself through another's eyes can be deeply shaming or profoundly healing. I have created a kind of theatre for shy people, a place where they can be seen and heard, with the deep knowing that they will be able to step onto the stage and at the same time step into the next stage in their lives. I have developed a process for directing *self-revelatory performance* (Self-Rev) that I term the *Embodied Life Stories Process*. This chapter explores the structures and the theoretical framework of this process by addressing how to access story from the body, when to use writing, when to improvise, when to witness, and how to find the deeper story.

The role of the self-revelatory director as the first witness can mirror the attachment of early childhood. The role of the audience as witness can repair a vital link, bringing the person back into community from isolation. The act of unpacking stories, first to the self-revelatory director, then to the audience, can be profoundly healing and transforming. Each story in our lives is like a pebble splashing into the pond of our inner worlds,

S. Rubin (✉)
Private Practice, San Francisco and Berkeley, CA, USA

JFK University, Department of Somatic Psychology, Pleasant Hill, CA, USA
e-mail: sheilarubin@sbcglobal.net

S. Pendzik et al. (eds.), *The Self in Performance*,
DOI 10.1057/978-1-137-53593-1_9

129

creating ripples that flow outward into the rest of our being. When there has been trauma, the stories that would have naturally flowed outward can get truncated, withheld, or lost. The level of support and attunement between the self-revelatory director and the storyteller/improviser can create a safe-enough container for the student to step out of shame and feel and express his or her true self.

For the facilitator directing a Self-Rev, each meeting with the student is a piece of sacred work in which the facilitator takes on roles of drama therapist, guide, director, parent, shaman, priestess, cheerleader, or trickster. I first ask students what their vision is and then lead them through a drama therapy process involving a series of improvisations and writing practices that create an embodied experience of their life stories. What emerges at deeper and deeper levels and with amazing complexity are their coherent life narratives as they create their Self-Rev. The process is much like the process of gestation and birth in the creating of the client's self. Sometimes the work is on a one-to-one basis and sometimes it is in a group format. The individual work has largely been with students in the Drama Therapy Program at the California Institute of Integral Studies who are completing their Self-Rev process as a capstone project. The group work has been my ten or twelve-week Embodied Life-Stories groups for members of the community.

Working with Trauma and Shame

The Self-Rev process can help traumatized individuals put the many parts of their lives back together. Here is one example: Early in the second rehearsal of an individual Self-Rev I am directing, the student begins to tell her story and then just stops. I touch her shoulder from a little behind her; we are both looking forward, across the room, as if this were a performance. I speak a few lines, continuing to tell her story, and stop. Then she begins and stops. Her story unfolds slowly this way. I am *co-teller* and a witness. I am slowing down the process. I am stepping into her silence and adding words. The back and forth of the telling creates a container. The aesthetic distance holds her process. At one point she names the abuse and her words stop. A few moments of silence pass as I let myself fully 'feel into' what she is sharing. Words float up for me to say: 'And I didn't know what to do,' I add. She cries, turns around and looks at me. 'This is the first time I've ever told anyone about what really happened, about the abuse.' We cry together.

I create a loving environment and offer witnessing, so the person who is struggling with shame can experience being supported and cared for. I am creating attachment through my witnessing, which starts from the first moment: being seen in a positive way, which is counter-shaming. I am working back and forth with several of the seven levels of witnessing (described below), much like a dance of attachment and distancing. I adjust based on what is needed in the moment, which leads to deeper material, or a safe place.

Renée Emunah (1994, 2015) writes about Self-Rev as a process that transforms painful material—something that is on a person's psychological edge, that perhaps he or she wants to move forward but doesn't know how—into art. She sees Self-Rev as a new kind of therapy and a form of theater that builds on the works of Grotowski, Artaud, The Living Theater, and other theater directors and companies. She says that in order to be riveting, the personal must also be universal.

Landy (1986), writing about aesthetic distance, explains that the over-distanced person may be blocking the experience from being felt, and the underdistanced person may be overwhelmed by painful emotional experience. The drama therapist guides gently in the needed direction until aesthetic distance is met with a deep realization, a sigh of relief or some tears. Kohut (1990) explains how deficits in a person's need for mirroring, idealization, and twinship—concepts from self-psychology—can be worked with in therapy. Through the self-revelatory process I am describing in this chapter, we restore the interpersonal bridge that Kaufman (1974) says is broken and heal the shame while creating a coherent narrative. We are nurturing and supporting the person through a deeply personal and transformative journey. Kaufman (1974) provides an early theory of shame development and resolution:

> Shame is a primary affect that is induced interpersonally. Shame inducement occurs when one significant person breaks the interpersonal bridge with another. Following internalization of shame within the personality, shame activation becomes an autonomous function of the self and the sense of shame lies at the core of one's identity as a person. Therapy needs to aim at dis-internalizing shame, enabling the client to effectively cope with the sources of shame without internalizing that affect, and enabling the client to affirm himself [or herself] from within. Most importantly, within the therapeutic relationship, the therapist needs to return internalized, autonomous shame to its interpersonal origins, thereby reversing the developmental sequence. (pp. 1–2)

When we become significant to another person, as happens when we are therapist, supervisor, friend, partner, spouse, or parent, then we can induce shame in him or her unconsciously or unintentionally, often without knowing it has happened. Failure to fully hear and understand the other's need and to communicate its validity—a look in the other direction, a frown, a disappointing facial expression—can sever the bridge and induce shame. Developmental needs that are not met over time can also lead to internalized shame. The child learns to feel shame that his or her needs do not matter; the rupture is from outside, from the parent who fails to validate the child's needs. This kind of shame leads to ruptures in the family, which in turn culminate in ruptures within the self, from the interpersonal to the intrapersonal domain. Kaufman (1974) proposes that counter-shaming experiences (e.g., acknowledging strengths of the client or similarities that the client has with the therapist) can restore the interpersonal bridge. Many exercises in the first two phases of Renée Emunah's *Integrative Five Phase model* of drama therapy (1994, 2009) provide counter-shaming experiences as they build self-worth through a series of successes. Many of the students with whom I work feel that 'something is wrong with me.' Many are filled with shame without knowing why.

LIFE STORIES: FINDING THE DEEPER STORY

I am guiding the person to find the deeper story. We are finding threads and themes that work with paradox, family history, and what participants think is their life story. I am looking for where there is act hunger—where there is a scene or part of a scene that wants to be seen or grown. The deeper story is found when a person digs deep enough in the right places that they come upon an underground river of archetypal human themes, allowing authenticity and creativity to spring forth (Rubin, 2007, 2015).

Metzger (1992) writes that stories heal us because we become whole through them. She says that in the process of writing we discover our story by restoring those parts of ourself that have been scattered, denied, distorted, or hidden and that stories heal through our remembering and integrating parts of ourselves. Landy (1993) writes that a role needs a story in order to communicate its essence, and that stories provide a container within which to work with roles. Gersie (1991) writes that stories provide a process through which we give form to our life, give voice to our inner experience, and shed light on the contrast between inner and outer worlds. Johnson (1991) notes that dramatic enactment is a process of creating something from nothing and transforming suffering into art.

LEVELS OF WITNESSING AND STORY

There are seven levels of witnessing to which I attend when I direct Self-Revs. These different levels relate to the attachment-related safety and security that are needed before genuine self-expression can begin. These levels relate to developmental attachment phases of early parent–child relationships: 'I see you', 'I hear you', 'I feel you', 'I understand you', 'Tell me more', 'Is this too much?' and 'I'm curious about_____.'

Even though a story has a beginning, middle and an end, where we begin the story can make all the difference. What we include in it this time is different than it would have been five minutes ago or next week. We can move back and forth in time to different levels of story, perspectives, and voices. We can discover and uncover the deeper story that touches a personal thread as well as universal or archetypal themes. There are many different types of stories: personal, family, community stories; embodied, mythic, spiritual, religious, stories; archetypal, historical, symbolic stories. The telling of stories can consist of dreams, masks, objects to represent parts of a person's family, inner world, psyche, family dynamics, psycho-drama, or inner roles. The story may be about parts of the person at a different age, each with its unique act hunger. The story may be the victim story, the healing story, the old story, or the next story. Often these stories emerge in the free-writing we do between improvisation sessions. The free-writing allows distance from the recent storytelling or improvisational process. When I notice the student's or group's hesitation just before an impasse, I often introduce an exercise to help them through it. David Johnson's *Developmental Transformations* (Johnson, 1982) provides improvisational interventions that I find helpful in working with story at these times: *faithful rendering* where the client just tells the story as is; *act completion* invites the story to be completed in ideal or tragic trajectories that can be exaggerated and explored; *defining* what really happened or where they are stuck in this story; *repetition*, where words, sounds, or movements in the story are repeated: *intensification*, asking the client to intensify various dramatic elements of the story; *joining* with them so we are both exploring the same moment in the story, or agreeing with them; *bracketing*, framing parts of the story in special ways; and *transformation to the here and now*, where we shift from being within a disturbing part of their story to witnessing it from the present.

The Self-Revs I direct involve a first phase of improvisation and free-writing, followed by weeks of script development. The self-revelatory narrative that may evoke fear, anxiety, helplessness, or shame can be tolerated in the safety of the present, and differentiated from the past. The person can learn to relate to these dreaded states differently. Actions that could not be taken can now be chosen (e.g., being able to run away from or confront a hurtful adult). New neural integrations may be formed throughout the brain and nervous system during this transformative experience of revising embodied stories. In *The Body Remembers*, Rothschild (2000) writes that *somatic memories* of frightening traumatic events can be transformed by connecting them with forgotten resources living in current body sensations.

This corrective emotional experience is further supported by rebuilding the interpersonal bridge between the person and the audience in the performance (Kaufman, 1974). Emunah (1994) writes that the performers' responses are exhilaration, pride, and the affirmation of identity. In contrast to traditional theatre, where the applause is for the actor's performances, in Self-Rev, the applause is for the person themselves. They are applauded for the courage to reveal themselves. The response of the audience demonstrates their acceptance of the performer and what they have lived through.

Example 1: The Go Button

An unemployed teacher attending my embodied life-stories group said she was coping with depression after not working for a year. She said, 'I'm stuck and can't move at all, my voice is frozen.' I worked with her depression and shame, first by normalizing it and inviting her to move slowly without judgment. Then I interviewed her depression:

'So, how long have you been with Mary Jo?'
'A long time!'
'What do you do for her?' I ask.
'I keep her safe!' says Depression, loudly.
'How do you keep her safe?'
'By keeping her tired and stuck.'
'How come?'
'If she's depressed, she won't make any stupid mistakes.'
'Oh, so you don't want her to make any mistakes. What kind of mistakes are you trying to stop her from making?'
'Every time she gets a job interview, I know she's going to get her hopes up.'

'So you don't want her to be disappointed,' I say.

'Exactly.'

'So if she's depressed, you're keeping her from making a mistake and hoping for something that might not happen.'

I then invite Mary Jo to do a one-minute improvisation to explore the role of depression. Depression says, 'She's too sensitive. It's my job to make sure she stays stuck because that's what I know. That's what she's always known.' I have Mary Jo do some free-writing about times she's been depressed, then about times she found a way out of depression. During one of the free-writing exercises she remembers being a youth camp participant working with a scared lamb. I ask her to find one movement she used to soothe the lamb. She starts petting the lamb.

As we play, I invite her to improvise slowly petting the lamb and moving around the room; I'm trying to help her to unpack the story. 'This lamb is safe at home,' she says. 'I took it to the fair and it wouldn't come off the truck. I kept sitting there and didn't know what to do.' Step by step we retrieve pieces of the story. She suddenly remembers a kind adult who asked her about her lamb and if it was her first time at the fair. 'This person taught me where the "go button" was on the lamb. If I pressed there, the lamb followed me everywhere!'

I was helping Mary Jo find the embodied stories of her life. Eventually she found the 'go button' from a childhood sheep competition and started to joyfully move the sheep around the room faster and faster. I watched as her body came out of that frozen, stuck place and witnessed delight, amazement, and excitement in her face and voice. As Mary Jo's stories deepened, she added more relational elements. She had had a dream about a drawer where she kept her feelings. 'Can you show me?' I asked. She pulled the drawer open and slowly closed it. I invited her to explore the image further: 'I remember my mother... I was her favorite... she loved me... I was so little... my parents separated... suddenly my dad took me and never brought me back to her... He wanted to hurt her... but it hurt me... no one to talk to... this is where I put all my feelings!'

I ask what she needs to hear from the audience. 'That it's okay to have these feelings!' At the performance, she asks the audience this question and the audience responds, 'Yes!!!!' Various audience members shout: 'Your feelings are your feelings!' 'You have a right to them!' 'We want to hear your feelings!' She moves her hand to open the drawer and pours out the pain, loneliness, and shame of feeling so alone all these years. The audience witnesses Mary Jo as she lets out the feelings and improvises. There is cheering. She cries and laughs and empties out the drawer by turning it upside down. There is much life force in her compared to a few weeks ago. The audience's loving witnessing and validating support can take her healing yet another level deeper. Now she is not cut off and isolated, but can bring more of herself forward. She finds not only safety, but also acceptance, caring, understanding, encouragement, and energy in community. Shame and despair fade.

Three months after our embodied life-stories performance, Mary Jo let me know that she had used the energy of the performance to get a job.

Example 2: Working from the Body

In *The Body Remembers*, Rothschild (2000) writes about ways that the body holds trauma and refers to safe ways to carefully work with trauma from a somatic perspective. In a life-stories workshop I was leading at a university, one teenage student found a way to process a profound and incomprehensible loss as I led a guided visualization: 'Rub your feet and let them remember shoes you've worn at different ages. When did you get your first running shoes? Sports shoes? Rubbing your feet and remembering sports as a kid... rubbing your ankle and remembering a comforting or fun physical activity you did as a young child... as a teen... as an adult...' The student read the free-writing that followed the visualization to the group. As he was remembering the pain in his foot, a memory of skating and skiing with best friend Joe surfaced. He remembered playing with Joe from childhood and into high school. They were always together until Joe was killed in a fight.

I led this student into an improvised movement exercise. He imagined the scene of the fatal fight his friend had been in. He found the movements of swinging the bat, throwing the baseball and the punch that a stranger had thrown—leading to falling to the ground and shoveling the dirt. He was able to do a movement sequence in which he correlated all the movements of baseball with his best friend's death. The response of the group was profound. He said later that he opened his eyes, saw their red eyes and heard cries. The story of his friend's death had been wrapped tightly in his embarrassment of not knowing how to talk about his loss. Telling the story in this embodied way helped him connect with the emotions that he had blocked. He unpacked his shock and shame and restored the interpersonal bridge as people reached out with their care and compassion.

This process helped him come to terms with the loss, with his own mortality, and with the shame of not knowing how to grieve. He was now able to begin the process of organizing these experiences into a coherent narrative as part of the Self-Rev process.

HEARING FROM THE AUDIENCE

I ask students what they need the audience to witness. Do they need a response? I help them to identify their needs and desires so as to shape their communicative narratives, and to increase the likelihood that their needs will be met through the process.

Here are some examples of what performers needed to hear from the audience:

- A woman in her 70s explores what 'sexy' means at each decade, and as a result reclaims her femininity and sacredness as a woman, and updates her vitality. The audience replies, 'You're still hot!' 'Can you teach a class on that?'
- A man titles his piece: 'Apologies float like a feather down to a deep pool, never arriving,' in which he shares how he was brutally teased in high school. The audience replies, 'We're so sorry.' 'They were cruel.'
- A neglected child is now an adult talking to a tape recorder, because there was no one to listen to them. The audience replies, 'We hear you now.'
- A woman has lost all of her family, and talks on stage about being the only one left. The audience shouts out, 'We're glad you're still here.'
- A woman tells a story she's never shared about an absolutely horrific event 'that there are no words for.' She asks that the audience not reply, just make eye contact, and they do, looking at each other for many minutes in intense silence.

The audience of a Self-Rev is here to participate in a healing ritual, not to be entertained. I invite the audience to close their eyes and feel the beating of their hearts, the power and the rhythm. Then I invite them to soften their hearts to receive the stories in the Self-Revs this evening. The students can see the eyes of the audience and hear how they are touched. Many audience members report being reminded of their own life experiences. There is often a feeling of universality and connectedness during and after the performance.

Hearing from the audience has been a vital part of my own Self-Rev performances and my graduate thesis *The role of the storyteller in self-revelatory performance* (1996)—given my memories of having my words consistently misunderstood by my mother, and having to create meaning in the world on my own. When there has been a big secret, when there has been profound dysfunction in a family, this performance process can allow a rebirth in which the person is held and witnessed in a new way. I needed witnessing of the story of how I grew up. I needed to share the story in a way that was compelling and that would elicit compassion and deep understanding. Using humor and distance via the role of the storyteller allowed me to step into and out of the trauma and shame from my childhood as the storyteller wove a coherent narrative. I needed to take the audience into my childhood home and hear their compassionate responses. That was very healing of my shame as I stepped out of the performance and into my professional identity as a drama therapist.

CONCLUSION

In directing Self-Revs, I am working to repair the interpersonal bridge that has been broken through shame in the person's history. We repair it first through their connection to me, then to members of the group, and finally to members of an invited audience to whom they tell their embodied life story. As this bridge heals through the witnessing, something happens to repair the damage done by the trauma to the person and their interpersonal relationships. Shame and the relentless negative thoughts about the self diminish, allowing the person to re-join others in a safer connection.

The work begins with the body to access stories through improvisational movement. When something emerges that may be painful or puzzling, I invite participants to do free-writing based on what emerged. The free-writing can release the inner critic and also spur the person into further exploration of the deeper story. Often we play with paradox. Each level of witnessing invites the person to take the story deeper. Themes and threads that have been invisible and disconnected emerge. There is now a way forward. The story that must be told is told and then witnessed, and the shame can be transformed. The audience is also touched, and may be reminded of their own stories and struggles. In the end, the message from audience to performer is simply and powerfully: 'You are amazing... Thank you for your story.'

REFERENCES

Emunah, R. (1994). *Acting for real: Drama therapy processes, technique and performance*. New York: Brunner-Mazel; Taylor & Francis.

Emunah, R. (2009). The integrative five phase model of drama therapy. In D. Johnson & R. Emunah (Eds.), *Current approaches in drama therapy* (2nd ed., pp. 37–64). Springfield, IL: Charles C. Thomas.

Emunah, R. (2015). Self-revelatory performance: A form of drama therapy and theatre. *Drama Therapy Review, 1*(1), 71–85.

Gersie, A. (1991). *Storymaking in bereavement: Dragons fight in the meadow*. London: Jessica Kingsley Publishers.

Johnson, D. (1982). The theory and technique of transformations in drama therapy. *Arts in Psychotherapy, 18*, 285–300.

Johnson, D. (1991). On being one and many. *Arts in Psychotherapy, 18*, 1–5.

Johnson, D. (1992). The drama therapist in role. In S. Jennings (Ed.), *Drama therapy: Theory and practice* (Vol. 2, pp. 112–136). London: Routledge.

Kaufman, G. (1974). *On shame, identity and the dynamics of change*. Lansing, MI: Michigan State University.

Kohut, H. (1990). *The search for self*. New York: International Universities Press.

Landy, R. (1986). *Drama therapy*. Springfield, IL: Charles C. Thomas.

Landy, R. (1993). *Persona and performance*. New York: Guilford.

Metzger, D. (1992). *Writing for your life: A guide and companion to the inner worlds*. New York: Harper Collins.

Rothschild, S. (2000). *The body remembers: The psychophysiology of trauma*. New York: Norton.

Rubin, S. (1996). *The role of the storyteller in self-revelatory performance*. Masters Thesis California Institute of Integral Studies. UMI Dissertation Services, Ann Arbor MI.

Rubin, S. (2007). Self revelatory performance. In A. Blatner (Ed.), *Interactive and improvisational drama: Varieties of applied theatre and performance* (pp. 250–259). New York: Universe.

Rubin, S. (2015). Almost magic: Working with the shame that underlies depression using drama therapy in the imaginal realm. In S. Brooke & C. Meyers (Eds.), *The use of the creative therapies in treating depression*. (pp. 231–244). Springfield, IL. Charles C Thomas.

CHAPTER 10

Restoried Script Performance

Pam Dunne

Defined as a live performance with aesthetic and personal elements, a *restoried script performance* (RS Performance) highlights a significant, relevant aspect of a person's life that has been restructured through a series of therapeutic processes. The restorying processes are informed by Narrative Therapy (White & Epston, 1990) and Narradrama (Dunne, 2006), and include the identification and enactment of *unique outcomes, healing stories*, and *problem-saturated stories*. The performance may be a solo piece, a collaborative script of collective personal stories, or a combination of poetry, video, dance, and/or monologue. Audiences may be personally connected to the performer or public. An RS performance is not a substitute for therapy, but the process and ultimate performance creates the possibility for transformation, self-discovery, and healing. This chapter will describe the RS performance process, examining the relevant theories and research that support its therapeutic benefits.

P. Dunne, PhD, RDT-BCT (✉)
California State University (Professor Emerita), Los Angeles, CA, USA

Drama Therapy Institute of Los Angeles, Santa Monica, CA, USA
e-mail: pdianedunne@hotmail.com

© The Author(s) 2016
S. Pendzik et al. (eds.), *The Self in Performance*,
DOI 10.1057/978-1-137-53593-1_10

141

NARRATIVE THERAPY

In Narrative Therapy, the act of *storying* is an integral self-organizing process that provides a means for reflection and discovering personal meaning (White, 2007). The *restorying* or re-authoring process, in turn, involves constructing a revised narrative embedded with new personal meaning and emotion that results from the experience of this process. The late Michael White, the leading international pioneer in Narrative Therapy, emphasized that 'the restorying of experience necessitates the active involvement of persons in the reorganization of their experience' (White & Epston, 1990, p. 13). Restorying clients identify new descriptions of their own identity and move from problem-saturated stories to alternative stories and unique outcomes. Unique outcomes (sometimes referred to as victory stories) are narratives in which a participant acts in her preferred way toward a problem within the story. Alternative stories present a more favorable picture of a participant. Unique outcome and alternative stories are both imperative in the restorying process, as they tend to produce positive emotions. Problem-saturated stories, on the other hand, often produce negative emotions because the problem and the negativity associated with that problem is still at the core of the narrative. In healing stories, narrative therapists utilize the techniques of externalization and scaffolding, a method of asking incremental questions, both of which can help participants discover possibilities of improving their present circumstances.

RS AND SELF-REVELATORY PERFORMANCE

While narrative therapy focuses on restorying processes that create new meanings through conversation and reflection, drama therapy allows for an integrated and embodied approach that creates new meanings through action. The performance aspect of an RS originates from theatre, but also shares some commonality with *self-revelatory performance* (Self-Rev) (Emunah, 2015). While both RS performance and Self-Rev aim for the transformation of the participant, the actual process and steps the participant embarks on to get there differ. Self-Rev performance is defined as a form in which a performer originates a theatre piece drawn from current life issues in need of healing (Emunah, 2015). One of the chief components of this approach is the concept of *working through* or working with. This means that there is a conscious effort on the part of the participant to contend with the material, which could entail confronting, shifting, embracing, or forgiving (Emunah, 2015). The idea is that through this process the participant will eventually arrive at a healthier state (ibid, 2015). While both RS performance and Self-Rev explore compelling personal issues, the RS performance focuses specifically on the process of re-scripting life stories.

In Self-Rev, the drama therapist working with a performer combines the roles of drama therapist and director. The director intervenes gently as the participant works through life challenges. In Self-Rev, 'the performer ultimately reaches for understanding, acceptance, validation, re-configuration, transformation, or mastery of the various parts of his/her psyche' (Emunah, 2015, p. 75). As the piece begins to emerge during the process of developing a Self-Rev, the director helps to hone theatrical awareness, ensuring that the piece will be one of artistic merit. In a RS performance, the drama therapist collaborates with the participant to integrate unique outcomes as well as new roles and identities, and serves as an active therapeutic support to the participant through each step of the restorying process and performance. The emphasis therefore is primarily on the therapeutic process while supporting the artistic merit of the theatrical performance.

Positive and Negative Emotion Research

The RS performance process is supported by a variety of research studies. Positive Psychology and Narrative Therapy research demonstrates the importance of positive emotions. When people feel good, their thinking becomes more creative, integrative, flexible, and open to information. Even though positive emotions are often short-lived, they can have deep, enduring effects. By momentarily broadening attention and thinking, positive emotions can lead to the discovery of novel ideas, actions, and social bonds (Fredrickson, 2003). In two recent studies in which cardiovascular activity was monitored by sensors, it was confirmed that positive emotions help to reduce cardiovascular reactivity (Fredrickson et al., 2000). Positive emotional states also affect heart rate variability, harmonious synchronization of beats (coherence), body connectedness (optimal body performance), as well as brain entrainment (in which the brain follows the patterns of the heart).

Positive affect has been shown to reinforce preferred outcomes and behaviors. Research in the field of Interpersonal Neurobiology confirms that as neural networks grow stronger in relationship to a new repetitive behavior, this new behavior is reinforced (Siegel, 2010). This is made possible by the strengthening of synaptic connections. While the neural network will remain 'thin' at first, through repeated neural linking and firing, it will progressively expand in thickness and connection speed (Siegel, 2012), which strengthens the likelihood that a new, restoried behavior will become the more dominant—and healthy—behavior.

Negative affect, on the other hand, contributes to negative effects on the body and mind, such as reducing blood flow to the frontal lobe (self-control and thinking part of the brain), reducing memory of peripheral information, increasing cortisol production, engaging the 'fight-or-flight' response, freeze system, as well as diminishing one's ability to connect. The effect of negative emotion is thought to be visible at both the cellular and structural level. When clients continuously struggle with issues of depression, anxiety, or anger, the experiences associated with these brain states get repeatedly reinforced. This limits the experience of other affective states (Grimm et al., 2009). During the RS Performance process, participants will undoubtedly encounter negative emotions, but with newly affirmed strengths, the participant doesn't get trapped or overwhelmed by these negative emotions and can move into preferred, positive affective states more easily.

Unique Outcomes and Narradrama Research

Leading researchers Marie-Nathalie Beaudoin and Jeffrey Zimmerman (2011) looked at the effects of increased emotion with regard to what they refer to as the *affect-infused unique outcome scene*. Their research confirmed that if the participant was encouraged to give a fuller, detailed description of the *where*, *when*, and *what*, the result was an increase in the emotional arousal of that participant (usually positive emotion) as well a more prominent engagement during the process itself. They used the narrative method of scaffolding, or incremental interview questions, to elicit a more detailed description from the participant—and found this to be helpful (White, 2007). Results indicated that affect increased both on the experiential and physiological levels. Bringing forth feelings and details about the experience rendered preferred-identity conclusions more accessible (Beaudoin & Zimmerman, 2011).

Savage (2013, 2015) conducted two studies in Narradrama focusing specifically on unique outcomes, with adolescent boys and girls in an adoption program and in a process drama and performance project. Qualitative analysis indicated that the participants successfully redefined and reconstructed their personal narratives in preferred and positive ways, supporting their personal growth and self-esteem, consistent with the findings of Beaudoin & Zimmerman (2011).

THE RESTORIED SCRIPT PROCESS

A RS process requires extended preparation and processing time for participants to fully explore aspects of themselves, including their stories, conflicts, journeys, and dreams. Restorying provides the participant the opportunity to create and mark new identity descriptions, inspired ideas, preferred views of stories, and successful victories over their problems. By expanding restoried outcomes, participants come to understand and confirm their newly discovered strengths.

The restorying process brings to the fore moments in the life of the participant that demonstrate personal agency. To further expand the implications of the scene, the therapist-director may interview the participant 'in role' as herself or another character in the scene, either by pausing the scene or after the conclusion of the scene. The interview focuses on identifying positive strengths and actions in various moments in the scene. These moments, in turn, provide a new way of constructing self-identity, recognizing strengths, appreciating parts of oneself, and finding new solutions to problems, which furthers the development of the RS performance.

While new meaning occurs during enactment, further meanings may continue to be developed through interviewing and reflecting about the moment, thereby strengthening changed identity, agency, and the effects of unique outcome and healing scenes. Meaning attribution may be assisted by open-ended therapeutic questions such as: 'In what way do you think these discoveries might affect your attitude toward yourself?' and 'What does your ability to move forward say about you as a person?' Meaning can also be ascribed through journal writing, drawing, and interviewing the participant 'in role.'

Participants are then encouraged to explore the idea of their new futures. These explorations are ascribed to their changed identity, as well as to the development of personal agency, and may be expanded through questions, such as: 'With the steps you've taken so far in the moment how does this contribute to the way you see yourself and what you value?' Or 'As a result of these steps, what different possibilities could occur in your future?' Possibility maps, which involve drawing a map in a preferred way and using map symbols to represent new possibilities, can be helpful at this stage to inform a progression in a RS performance. Preferred future scenes may also be performed. Often future scenes become an integral part of the script.

As the drama therapist prepares to move into the first step toward the RS performance, the underlying restorying structure suggested above needs to be facilitated within the following three steps to solidify and mark these important moments.

Step 1: Pictorial History

In the first step, the participant draws a pictorial history of significant scenes in their life (at least ten pictures, from birth to the present). The participant chooses the drawing style with which they are most comfortable, such as sketching, or the use simple stick figures or symbols. In small groups, participants share and perform living sculptures that are like still photos which can then be examined and reflected upon. Various narrative focal points are used to create the living sculpture, such as preferred drawings, emotionally compelling drawings, or a blank paper, which represents a scene they would like to see. A binder holds these pictures so others can be added throughout the development of their restoried script. Often in pictorial dramatizations, a healing story or a unique outcome might emerge from one of the drawings, or in the blank drawing, which leads easily into Step 2.

Step 2: Narrative-Focused Warm-Ups

Narrative warm-ups aid the participant in discovering new ways to look at their own stories and roles within those stories, with special attention given to moments and roles that reveal strengths and personal agency. It is often during this step that participants discover a theme, pattern, or idea that will ultimately shape the nature of their RS performance. Three examples of narrative-focused warm-ups are discussed below: healing stories, unique-outcome stories, and self-role monologues.

Healing Stories
A healing story is a nonfictional narrative in which the participant experiences positive emotions—such as love, security, warmth, affection, and trust—towards, and from, a significant other. In the example below we

meet Jing, a young Japanese woman who left her country and her history of abuse, to claim a new life in the USA. Her father, who died when she was 12, is the subject of her healing story.

> When I was a little girl, my father taught me a haiku. It was about a morning glory. The rope for the well bucket is taken over by a morning glory vine, and that person doesn't want to cut the vine or take the rope away from that morning glory. So she goes next door to ask for the water. So the morning glory can stay where it's comfortable. My father said he wanted me to be like that person, a kind person. On the way back home from school, I noticed some sparrows drinking water from a puddle of water ahead. I stopped and watched them drink water. I thought of the morning glory haiku my father taught me. I didn't want to scare the sparrows away. They wanted to drink water. So I waited there and watched them drink water, until a car drove by and scared them away. When I got home, my father was waiting for me, all worried. I didn't realize I was watching sparrows for that long! I told him, 'I'm sorry, Daddy, I had to wait for the sparrows to finish drinking water.' That made him smile. He knew that I was trying to be kind like he told me to. He was happy. And I was happy, too, because I made him happy...

Unique Outcome Stories

A healing story sometimes provides a path to a unique outcome story because the benefits experienced by the healing story can create a safer, more restorative place for the participant to explore from. A unique outcome story reflects a scene from the participant's life in which she acts in her preferred way toward a problem. Unique outcome stories move the process of the RS forward, as the participant begins to internalize the exercise work, becoming cognizant of the new, preferred descriptions she is developing and performing in the exercise. This work ultimately reveals her preferred ways of being in relationships, responses toward problems, and in pursuing the future she desires, all of which often provide the basis of her RS. In the excerpt below, Farhad, an educated male in his 50s who has battled ADHD throughout his life, explores other aspects of himself through two songs: one that represents a problem-saturated moment, and another more positive unique outcome moment.

> Ah, not that song again. That's not the song I'm trying to remember, it's too sad. I don't mean sad, it's cold. (He hums a tune). Tatatata.

Gole-yakh-tuye dellam javuneh kardeh (Translation: 'Ice flowers blooming in my heart).'

I mean, I love the image of flowers blooming. But these lyrics are about wallowing in self-pity, losing heart, losing compassion. I'm trying to remember that other song, a warm song that inspired me. It's by the same singer, Kourosh, from the late 60s, or early 70s. I was 13–14 years old, lived in Iran, when a new kind of Persian music was being born. I used to dance with Jacqueline at school parties (big smile), you know... I was going through puberty... And I would pour on the cologne, blow dry my hair, and put on those hi-hee... Leather boots. (BIG SMILE)... To dance with Jacqueline. Jacqueline and I were in love one day, and then we just fell out of love so quickly. (Whistling): tatatata. Wish I could remember that other song. It was not cold, not disheartened, It was a warm song, a hopeful song, a wise song...

Self-Role Monologues

Externalizing and performing a problem in a story through the self-role monologue exercise offers the participant the opportunity to uncover a clearer picture of the influence of a preferred role in her life. Self-role monologues may also be videotaped and played back for further reflection. In the example below, Gemma, a young woman who struggles with depression, created four short monologues to explore different roles. Excerpts from two of her four monologues explore the roles of Tara, an existing problem-saturated character, and Ariel, a new role that celebrated life.

Tara: I'm afraid of going, as I go to the dark place. Then sadness calls me like a sweet twisted nostalgia. I am a divided person. There's something down there that wants to suck me in. It's a force like gravity, pulling me down...

Ariel... Ladies and gentlemen, you are honored to be here today to listen to me because I am completely special and unique and also legendary...

Step 3: Creative Arts Exploration

The third step of the RS performance focuses on creative arts exploration exercises, which invite participants to perform moments of their story through art, music, drama (e.g., fairytale, contemporary story, myth), poetry, dance and photography/video (for examples of exercises, see Dunne, 2006). All of these forms integrate well with action techniques and provide opportunities for projection and emerging themes as the process deepens. Through short performances, participants explore the language of each art form and begin forming and refining their RS for their ultimate performance. Below are some examples of the use of various creative arts exercises in performance.

Example 1

A group of homeless and marginalized women drew masks of their externalized selves and their preferred selves. Some of the masks and themes appeared in their RS performance of *Rock Paper Scissors* and powerfully communicated their newly discovered identities to the audience, revealed in the following lines: 'I have a dream. It is the color of me', 'I can easily be my masterpiece root to leaf and petal to tree,' and 'I am an unfinished work of art' (Savage, 2015).

Example 2

A woman named Lynn used poetry to express the importance of advocacy in her piece:

> I will speak
> I will stand
> I will ferociously insist
> I will be relentless and true
> I will be for you
> I will ask only one thing, one thing in return
> I will ask you to teach me, teach me, as if I were your own...

Example 3

In Jing's restorying process, she continued to expand on her emerging themes of abuse and transformation, via a poem she wrote, entitled *Sinking*.

> ... Let go of the chain
> You would never know
> The sun always shines
> Above the thick clouds
> The sun always shines
> If you don't let go of the chain
> You would never know

The sun always rises
Beyond the gloomy sundown
The sun always rises...

In part, Jing's poem speaks to the abuse she endured at the hands of her brother and her fortitude to push ahead into a preferred present. Jing reflects: 'Let go, Let go of the chain, is the voice I finally found in myself.'

Example 4
Jing also creatively engaged in a personal song-writing exercise, and noticed how her theme of transformation emerged in her original song, entitled *Never Still*:

> ... But the nightmare is fading
> Your tears became the ocean
> Water is never still
> Let your hair melt in the air

After the performance of her song, Jing reflected, 'The water symbolism in the lyrics is very significant for me. Water never stays in one place or in one form—it keeps evolving. Transformation and fluidity keeps me moving and growing.'

Example 5
Charlotte, a graduate student, mother, wife, and full-time professional, explored her current life challenges via an exercise called *Self-Commercial*, reflecting:

Long shot of industrial soundstage with dancers. Hip music in the background (something by Moby or Groove Armada). We see a collage of hip and funky folks in cool duds dancing to the groove in an industrial setting. CAMERA PANS and Charlotte stands center on a sound stage, multi-colored lights and strobe dancing around her image.
CLOSE-UP: She is moving to the beat. A sultry female voice-over (ala Brenda Vaccaro) ANNOUNCES:
Mother Earth's 2015 model CHARLOTTE has arrived!
The newest mother-wife-student professional SUV is shining bright!
For freeway or dirt roads—any terrain will do.

Anti-lock system—always on alert for those marital, parental, and professional needs.

Ease your spirits—Don't test drive the CHARLOTTE—just go for it! You won't be disappointed!

Charlotte later reflected: 'I was the director, writer and actor! It was not just on the page, it ended up on a screen for others to see—to be witnessed. I focused on getting this message of motherhood and the complexities of juggling, which actually ran deeper than I thought as a problem.'

Example 6

Jing danced to a piano improvisation based on the song, *Over the Rainbow*, played by Keith Jarrett. The phrase 'somewhere over the rainbow' appeared later in conversation between Jing and the little girl in her RS performance. She slowly looked up as if to reach for something hopeful. In reflecting on the piece, Jing stated:

> I knew the musical and the song as a child. I remember the ending of my performance being very powerful and exhilarating. My movement suggested flying, reaching up and extending far. My wishing and longing transformed into confidence, and ability to see possibilities and hope to move forward in life.

RESTORIED SCRIPT PERFORMANCE

The ultimate RS performance is a culmination of all the refined scenes, themes, and new identities that emerge during the extensive process work. Performances range anywhere from 10 minutes to 45 minutes, and can be performed in a variety of forms, from a musical comedy to a poetic reading, from an opera to a multi-media performance. It is essential that the theatrical format accurately match the performer's vision.

Setting and Venue

Sometimes a traditional theater space is ideal because the stage can be set according to the participant's vision. However, participants may also decide that a site-specific location is optimal. For example, in one of the RS performances during a workshop I was teaching in Barcelona in 2010, participants chose various locations around the city, such as public parks and street corners, to perform their restoried scripts. One participant, Barbara, chose the subway as her ideal location, because of the flux of people and constant motion. Following is one of her fellow participants reflecting on that performance:

> The other players and I followed Barbara to witness her performance, which began while she was walking in the underground subway station. The main part of the drama took place on the subway. Barbara got on an adjoining car and began talking to a passenger. We all stayed in a connected car with a window observing. She confronted other people on the car and when getting off, her script continued while walking out of the subway and onto the street.

Audience

During a RS performance, the audience is not only viewing a work of art unfolding before them, but also being witnesses to a transformation. The audience is already keenly aware that no line exists between the performer and her role. There is an inherent connectedness between the audience and the performer, wherein support of the performer's courage, openness, and journey begins before the first line of her script.

Immediately following the performance, the RS performer(s) come out to meet the audience, who usually are a mix of family, friends, teachers, therapists, fellow RS participants, and the public. This is followed by a Q&A discussion, which affords the audience an opportunity to reflect with the participant about the performance they just witnessed. The Q&A most often takes the form of an open conversation between the two; however, sometimes the therapist-director may open with a warm-up and/or may encourage small groups (or pairs) to share their feedback. During the Q&A, there are often tearful exchanges between the audience and performer. Participants and audiences both value the Q&A, as the performer can reflect on how s/he felt understood, seen, and honored, and the audience members, in turn, can continue to learn about the participant. Answering audience questions also invites the performer to continue to reflect.

CONCLUSION: JING'S PERFORMANCE

Jing's final RS performance, entitled *Embrace*, was a wonderful example of personal transformation and restorying. Both her original song and poem, which were the outcome of her narrative-focused warm-ups, made their way into her final script as key parts of her story of courage and determination to move ahead despite her abusive past. Jing wrote her final RS performance script in lyrical form and sang beautifully throughout her 15-minute performance, her script alive with drive, compassion, and honesty. She concluded with this beautiful, healing image:

> The blue air is waiting
> Your fears became the melting snow
> Water is never still
> Let your hair dance in the air

As Jing sang this last line, and danced, with open arms outstretched towards the sky, the lights began to fade. In reflecting on her piece, Jing said:

> I remember crying as I wrote it. I feel the tears coming up as I reflect on this now… I feel that I was able to accept the reality and care for the little girl inside of me because of all this work.

The RS process and performance are vehicles that not only propel the participant forward in their life and preferred identity, but also that honor the person, along with his or her journey and ultimate transformation. As Jing writes,

> … The setting sun is also a rising sun if seen from the other side. The sense of hope I felt at this moment was truly amazing. So the poem and script is a message to my adolescent self, and to the little girl in me who still likes to sit in the swing and sing sometimes: choices and possibilities exist, and the sun always rises.

REFERENCES

Beaudoin, M. N., & Zimmerman, J. (2011). Narrative therapy and interpersonal neurobiology: Revisiting classic practices, developing new emphases. *Journal of Systemic Therapies, 30*(1), 1–13.

Dunne, P. (2006). *Narrative therapist and the arts* (2nd ed.). Los Angeles: Possibilities Press, an Imprint of the Drama Therapy Institute of Los Angeles.

Emunah, R. (2015). Self-revelatory performance: A form of drama therapy and theater. *Drama Therapy Review, 1*(1), 71–85.

Fredrickson, B. L. (2003). The value of positive emotions. *American Scientist, 91*(4), 330–335.

Fredrickson, B. L., Mancuso, R. A., Branigan, C., & Tugade, M. M. (2000). The undoing effect of positive emotions. *Motivation & Emotion, 24*(4), 237–258.

Grimm, S., Ernst, J., Boesiger, P., Schuepbach, D., Hell, D., Boeker, H., & Northoff, G. (2009). Increased self-focus in major depressive disorder is related to neural abnormalities in subcortical-cortical midline structures. *Human Brain Mapping, 30*(8), 2617–2627.

Savage, M. (2013). Using the self-commercial with adolescents in an adoption support services program: A narrative study. Published Dissertation, UMI Number 3706869, Ann Arbor, Michigan: Pro Quest LLC.

Savage, M. (2015). Re-storied script in game girls: Rock, paper, scissors. *Performance project based on the film Game Girls'* by filmmaker Alina Skrzeszewska.

Siegel, D. (2010). *Mindsight*. New York: Random House.

Siegel, D. (2012). *The developing mind (2nd ed.): How relationships and the brain interact to shape who we are*. New York: W.W. Norton.

White, M. (2007). *Maps of narrative practice*. New York: W.W. Norton.

White, M., & Epston, D. (1990). *Narrative means to therapeutic ends*. New York: W.W. Norton.

CHAPTER 11

The Performative: Life-Changing Moments in Autobiographical Performance

Gideon Zehavi

The *performative* is that moment in performance in which a transformation takes place in the experience of performer and audience members (Austin, 2007). These intersubjective, one-time and spontaneous moments are by no means guaranteed; they cannot be willed, do not always happen in the same instance or for the same duration, nor do they always arouse the same affective experience. This chapter delineates a three-phase structure that supports the emergence of performative moments in Autobiographical Performances: (1) an individual and introspective *preliminary phase*; (2) a *preparatory process*, wherein performatives occur between the director and performer; and (3) a *performance phase*, in which performatives take place between performer and audience.

Daniel Stern and other members of the Boston Change Process Study Group examined the central role of the *present moment* in change processes (Stern, 2004; Tronick, 1998). Stern defined present moments as unique and emotionally laden moments of encounter and transformation. The Boston CPSG examined moments of encounter and reciprocal exchange between infant and caregiver, as well as therapist and client,

G. Zehavi, MA, RDT-BCT (✉)
Hebrew University of Jerusalem, Jerusalem, Israel

Tel Hai Academic College, Kiryat Shmona, Israel
e-mail: gideon_zehavi@hotmail.com

© The Author(s) 2016
S. Pendzik et al. (eds.), *The Self in Performance*,
DOI 10.1057/978-1-137-53593-1_11

on small-scale time units, several seconds in length. These moments are mostly nonverbal, emotionally charged, intersubjective and potentially transformative (Stern, 2004). Stern differentiated between three present moment subtypes: (a) a *regular present moment*; (b) a *now moment* that is an emotionally-laden moment with an immediate potential for action and change; and (c) a *moment of meeting* that is intersubjectively experienced by two parties. Stern acknowledged that these small-scale units 'can be strung together and assembled into overarching units' (ibid., p. 149), thus making the present moment perspective applicable to *APs*.

Stern (2004) referred to the process of arriving at present moments as a *moving along process*. It is an unpredictable and sloppy process of two minds, conceivably director and performer, working to meet each other in a 'hit-miss-repair-elaborate' fashion (p. 156). He further states that in it '[…] they co-create islands of fittedness from the sloppiness [… and] forge larger spaces of shared implicit relational knowing' (p. 164).

The moving along process strongly corresponds to the preparatory process in the director–performer alliance and lays the foundations for performative moments to take place. In turn, preparatory processes contribute to the formation of shared representational structures that may emerge in performance. Performatives are those extraordinary, memorable and potentially life-changing intersubjective moments in autobiographical performances that audiences remember and value.

The findings that follow are based upon a comparative study of contemporary *autobiographical performances* (*AP*) and *drama therapy-based autobiographical performances* (*DTAP*). The former lie within the field of theatre and performance, while the latter holds an additional therapeutic intent and involve a director with drama therapy training, associated with what Renée Emunah (2015) has termed *self-revelatory performance* (Self-Rev). The results suggest that performative moments taking place in the second phase between the performer and director are necessary precursors to performatives in the performance phase.

Drama therapy-based autobiographical performances (DTAP) are postmodern in essence, as performers subjectively explore their life experiences as they grapple with issues of self identity, retrieve memories from their past, reconstruct life stories and present them before an audience. The performer attempts to balance representations of prior life events and the spontaneous unfolding of performatives in the moment. Emunah (2015) states that the intention of Self-Rev performance is to raise the psychological awareness of the performer, achieve therapeutic change and reveal something new to both performer and audience. Emunah (1994) differentiates between Self-Rev and other APs in that Self-Revs emerge from a drama therapy process, deal with the performer's current issues and entail a high level of emotional exposure and risk-taking. I prefer to use the term DTAP, however, as it highlights the use of drama therapy methodology, and is therefore more informative to the broader field of performance studies.

Drama therapy-based autobiographical performances are located within the fields of social theatre, drama therapy, and the larger field of performance studies. Social theatre is defined by James Thompson and Richard Schechner (2004) as 'theatre with specific social agendas; theatre where aesthetics is not the ruling objective' (p. 12). The two authors depict four groups of social theatre: (a) theatre for healing; (b) theatre for action; (c) theatre for community; and (d) theatre for transforming experience into art (p. 15), all closely related to *DTAPs*. *Aesthetic distance*, a point of balance between emotional expression and cognitive understanding (Landy, 1986), is key to the healing process in drama therapy and *DTAP* in particular.

In addition, *DTAP* is part of therapeutic theatre in drama therapy. Stephen Snow depicts therapeutic theatre as a rehearsal process and culminating performance developed with therapeutic intentions and goal-setting. Therapeutic theatre needs to be facilitated by a therapist skilled in drama or by a drama therapist; it is performed to community beyond the social sphere of the therapeutic group itself, and it consists of a post-production processing of the performance experience (Snow et al., 2003).

This chapter examines performatives in APs on three levels: (a) an overview locates *AP* within the fields of autobiography and performance studies and points out relevant concepts; (b) findings from a comparative study of four contemporary Israeli solo performances, consisting of two APs and two DTAPs, are reported. Performed from 2007 to the present, they were written by the performers and created with the support of outside directors. They were performed on numerous occasions before the general public with the intention of giving voice to untold experiences of violation and victimization; and (c) a concluding discussion examines the contribution of drama therapy and Daniel Stern's concept of the present moment to the understanding of autobiographical performances.

The Postmodern Performance

Since the second half of the twentieth century the phenomenon of performance has been extensively researched in many fields of social studies and the humanities. Irving Goffman (1959) broadly defined performance as 'all the activity of a given participant on a given occasion which serves to influence in any way any of the other participants' (p. 15). Schechner (2009) refers to performances as 'twice behaved behaviors,' that is, performed actions that people train for and rehearse (p. 28).

John Austin (2007) defined the term *performative* as 'performing actions' whereby in saying something a real action is carried out. He stated that in order for a performative to occur two conditions have to be met: (a) it has to be heard by someone; and (b) it has to be understood by him. Austin perceived performances that are not based in reality as false. However, many theoreticians and practitioners in the performing arts contested his view (Butler, 1988; Dolan, 2005; Grotowski, 1986) in that the stylized representations of life experiences in the performing arts are communicated by the performers to the audience and could have a real and sometimes life-changing effect on both parties.

In the 1960s, western theatre, in step with western arts, experienced a *performative turn* toward the postmodern (Fischer-Lichte, 2008). Theatrical events were no longer solely perceived as spectacles created and performed before an audience as objective works of art, but rather as subjective experiences that take place between performers and their audiences. Since the 1960s there has been a gradual shift of interest in theatre from the modernistic search for an essential truth to a postmodern 'lived experience' perspective. *DTAPs* made their debut in the early 1980s. The goal of reconstructing the performer's life story makes them postmodern in essence, yet they move back and forth between modern and postmodern aesthetic representations (Bailey, 2009; Du Rand, 1992).

In postmodern performances the boundaries separating the performance text from the performance, the performer from the performed, and all of the above from the audience, collapse to create a whole set of alternative dichotomies, such as aesthetic vs social, aesthetic vs political, and aesthetic vs ethical (Fischer-Lichte, 2008). In many APs and DTAPs, in particular, the performer seeks to move beyond the abstractions of modernism by returning to representational forms such as a reconstructed life story. The representational form, otherwise identified as the *neoconservative position* (Foster, 1984), characterizes the solo dramas reviewed in this chapter.

Autobiographical content is central to performing the self, carried out by the postmodern action of reassembling fragments of self, whether real or fantasized, into performance. Philippe Lejeune admitted that literary autobiography had nothing to do with an objective recounting of life events and was, therefore, essentially postmodern. He wrote:

Telling the truth about the self, constituting the self as complete subject—it is a fantasy. In spite of the fact that autobiography is impossible, this in no way prevents it from existing (1989, p. 131)

Jennifer Stephenson perceives twenty-first-century autobiographical performances as uniquely powerful political acts. She writes that '... through the invocation of performative power, it is possible to remake one's identity and write a new future or magically even a new past' (2013). She joins her feminist forerunner Judith Butler (1993) in stating that the contemporary autobiographical voice is available to women who have been excluded from the dominant discourse and whose stories have been dismissed as worthless.

The four solo performances in this study give voice to, and re-story, the performers' experiences of sexual abuse, domestic violence and potentially violating protocols of IVF treatments. The performers (three women and one man) explicitly expressed their conviction to share their life-stories with the public (Rubin, 2010).

THE PERFORMANCES

The four autobiographical performances studied were performed thirty or more times each before the general public in Israel from 2007 to the present. In the two DTAPs, the performer and director maintained a double focus on the performer's affective processes in conjunction with aesthetic considerations. In the two APs, the affective processes were not considered part of the preparatory structure. The following are brief outlines of the four performances:

Pshuta: Denuded (2007–2012). This AP was written and performed by Miki Peleg-Rothstein, directed by Norman Issa. A professional actress associated with *Habima*, the national theatre, Miki explicitly states that she decided 'to place her truth on stage' while accentuating aspects that are not part of her real-life experience (Jacobson, R., 2006). *Pshuta* holds multiple meanings: stripped bare (denuded), laid bare, a simple woman, and in Hebrew it has allusions to words like pussy and whip. This AP tells the story of Mira, a seven-year-old girl who suffers seven years of sexual abuse at the hands of her stepfather. Mira is daughter to a deaf mother who in her desperation seeks out another partner, remarries and turns her back on her two daughters. The dramatic text is delivered in the present tense. Mira shares with the audience parts of her diary, artistically staged sexual experiences, her inner rage, survival tactics, emotional deterioration to anorexia, multiple hospitalizations and culminating retribution.

Hasod Hagadol (The Great Secret) (2009–2012): This DTAP was written and performed by Maya Boltzmann, a psychodramatist, and directed by Osnat Schnek-Yosef, a theatre director and drama therapist. The performance deals with incest and Maya's journey in search of Mirta, her frozen inner child. Maya, the narrator of her childhood story, recounts the sexual abuse she experienced by her father as a small child in the basement of his pharmacy in Buenos Aires. Mirta had lost her memory, became socially disengaged, and eventually promiscuous. She did not die, but rather froze in time much like the child in Hans Christian Andersen's (1973) *Snow Queen.*

In performance Maya reconstructs her childhood memories with her siblings; represents her father's enchanting charisma; dares to symbolically climb down the basement steps to dramatically re-enact the trauma of incest; and in the aftermath reclaims Mirta and welcomes her back into her present life.

The Sad Tribe (2011–present): This DTAP was written and performed by Alex Vinegart, a professional actor and drama therapist and directed by Loscha Shimshoni, a professional director and Focusing practitioner. It is a DTAP dealing with immigration, fatherlessness and domestic violence set during the playwright's childhood. Alex plays the role of Moshe, a storyteller, who brings together two storylines: one of Misha, a child who emigrated to Israel without his father, who witnessed and suffered physical and emotional abuse from his stepfather and yet was able to take refuge in his gift for writing. The other is a self-created folktale of young Mobutu, an African youth, who searches for his tribe's lost sense of happiness. Alex Vinegart balances the enacted storylines with moments of mime and silence, pregnant with unspoken violence.

IV Yes or IV No: a Fertility Chart (2012–present): This AP was written and performed by Iris Harpaz, a professional actress and pianist and directed by Osnat Schnek-Yosef, a theatre director and drama therapist. An AP revealing the agonizing protocol and emotional turmoil the playwright/actor underwent in her In Vitro Fertilization (IVF) process, Liat Haim, the protagonist, tells the story of becoming a mother to Tsitsina, her unborn embryo. Undergoing IVF treatments, Liat Haim shifts back and forth from a cooperative and naïve perception of her fertility protocol to a disillusioned position regarding her chances of becoming a mother. Iris Harpaz strikes a fine balance between the bare facts of IVF protocol and the emotional rollercoaster ride Liat Haim experiences. She accompanies herself on piano to create a unique language combining music, physical theatre and text.

PHASES IN THE AUTOBIOGRAPHICAL PERFORMANCE PROCESS

Videotaped recordings and in-depth interviews held with the creators of the solo performances[1] are the basis of the study and its findings. Case examples illuminate important similarities and differences among the performances.

The Preliminary Phase

The initiation of an autobiographical process, that is, the moment the performer decides that s/he is embarking on a journey that will culminate in an AP, typically precedes the preparatory process and is highly individual and introspective. In three of the four performances studied the individual process began with the writing of a dramatic text.

Iris Harpaz relates that the writing process was sparked off by an IVF support group she attended. She remembers saying to the group that 'in the worst case scenario if I were not able have a child by treatment, I would at least have a play' (personal communication, 08/26/2014; Abramson, 2012). She recalls that '... on the morning after [the first meeting] I began to write the first monologue. [...It] brought out a lot from within and it made me feel really good, happy and calm' (ibid.). Amir Orian, an Israeli theatre theoretician, director and critic, mentored Iris through her preliminary writing process.

Miki Peleg-Rothstein states that writing the play 'was very intimate' (personal communication, 12/23/2014). It was a solitary process that took place in her son's bedroom wherein the computer was her only partner. She distinctly recalls that she '... did not deal with the things [she] would go through [in performance...] and did not imagine the audience' (ibid.).

Maya Boltzmann on the other hand acknowledges that the performance was never actually put into writing, even though the action had been set and rehearsed. She relates difficulties in memorizing texts to dissociative patterns linked to her traumatic experiences: '... several times we tried to write something, but it was no use... because many scenes and flashbacks suddenly came up' (personal communication, 12/17/2014).

The Preparatory Process

Forging the director–performer alliance is a first step in the preparatory process. Experiencing a sense of trust within the partnership was crucial in all four cases.

Miki Peleg-Rothstein initially directed herself in a 50-minute version of *Pshuta* and only after theatre repertoire committees critiqued her performance for being 'too harsh, 'in the face,' and 'volatile,' did she begin to search for an outside director (personal communication, 12/23/2014). Miki recalls the tension she experienced embarking on the joint process with Norman Issa and acknowledges that it was only after she let go of the playwright's position and committed herself solely to the actress role that she began to trust in Issa's directorial choices (ibid.).

Loscha Shimshoni likened her directorial work to a dance between the roles of director, choreographer and *Focusing* partner. The volatile materials Alex was grappling with were able to be contained and they both experienced a growing sense of family in the process (personal communication, 12/23/2014).

Turning Points

The four performers and their directors observed specific turning points in the preparatory process, occurring through the emergence of a form/language, a requirement in the staging, or a deepening in the director-performer alliance.

Alex Vinegart turned to the language of physical theatre and mime to express the numerous roles he embodied in performance. For instance, Alex mimed in slow motion the vindictive and displaced rage of Lenny, Misha's stepfather, as he turned over a tomato stand in a local market, or shattered the fish tank in the family's living room. Alex realized that the stylized representations of violence were better received by the audience in comparison to the realistic and vocal enactments that characterized the initial performances (personal communication, 10/2012).

Iris Hapaz and Osnat Schnek-Yosef agreed that the aesthetics of *IV Yes or IV NO* are based on a balance struck between Iris's stylized musical renditions and her use of physical theatre (personal communication, 08/26/2014). In a back and forth movement, Iris expressed irony, sarcasm and poignant self-revelation on piano alongside visceral enactments of her IVF treatments.

Maya Boltzmann and Osnat Schnek-Yosef made use of Hans Christian Andersen's *Snow Queen* fairytale as a basic structure and working metaphor. The lines Maya recites during the thrice-repeated rape scene were inspired by Andersen's (1973) text:

> *Somewhere in the sky/In the place where the harmful sprites dwell*
> *A terrible mirror shattered./Anyone who looked through it—*
> *Saw everything upside down./The good turned bad*
> *The beautiful turned ugly./The girl's heart froze into ice*
> *Unable to separate good from bad...*

Miki Peleg-Rothstein recalls that during their first rehearsal Norman Issa asked her to imagine playing with sand in her hands. The childlike metaphor was later expanded into a funnel-type prop that spewed out a steady stream of sand throughout the performance. The sand symbolized time, water, blood and semen and became Miki's inanimate stage partner (personal communication, 12/23/2014).

Osnat Schnek-Yosef notes that her work tends to revolve around a specific object (personal communication, 12/17/2014). In *The Great Secret* the object was a one-by-two meter solid pine wooden table placed center stage, symbolizing the pharmacy counter. Under this table, Maya re-enacted the basement rape scenes; and as she climbed, sat, stood and danced on it she represented Mirta's deteriorating and dissociative life.

Maya identifies that her sense of trust in Osnat was validated after they metaphorically descended the basement steps together and Osnat was able to stay present for her as she played out her childhood trauma for the first time (personal communication, 12/17/2014). Osnat also refers to the initial basement enactment as a milestone in the therapy process. Osnat states that they were able to reach a strong sense of embodied presence in a post-traumatic experience. She clarifies: '[When] we get to the critical points and allow ourselves to be present in our somatic experience... a sense of release is felt... Maya let herself reach a very deep somatic state, and even choked extensively... 'In that deep place I had to muster the confidence within me that her body knew what to do and that it will be okay in the end.... and [Maya] came to a place that she was never in before' (personal communication, 12/17/2014). Maya's basement experience deepened the sense of trust between the two, but, more importantly, it enabled her to achieve aesthetic distance in Osnat's presence. She was no longer left alone with *The Great Secret*, which erupted in recurring flashbacks and other overwhelming Post-Traumatic Stress Disorder (PTSD) symptoms. The enactment allowed her to feel the pain and looming danger, and at the same time to intentionally represent her trauma. Her experience was clearly communicated and transformed. She was able to shift away from the victim role, transition into the rehearsal process and aesthetically represent the rape sequences in the role of incest survivor. Ultimately, the aesthetic distance Maya achieved in the preparatory process enabled her to experience performative moments during the performance.

The Performance Phase

A performative moment in performance can frequently be traced back to performative moments within the director–performer alliance. For example, a key performative moment was reached in *The Sad Tribe* performance after Loscha Shimshoni, in spite of her aesthetic judgment, conceded to Alex's need to expand the role of Moshe, the storyteller, in order to gain aesthetic distance. The double focus held within the director–performer alliance between drama therapy-based processes and aesthetic considerations provided a framework wherein Loscha trusted that Alex's personal needs would be met within the aesthetics of performance. By emotionally distancing himself and enacting the rage and looming danger in the culminating scene from Moshe's adult perspective, Alex set the stage for the following performative moment:

> Alex, the actor, stands up, circles the chair and climbs on it. He takes on the role of Mobutu who had just returned from his journey to his tribe.
> Mobutu: Village folks, people of the Sad Tribe (short pause)… I have found our happiness. I, Mobutu, have found our lost happiness. Mother, father, my beloved brothers, come and see it is here in my hand (he points to his closed fist with his right hand).
> Moshe (storyteller): At that moment all the people gathered in the village square and looked at Mobutu who opened his hand and there they saw (short pause)… an empty hand. (Alex relaxes his stretched out hands and expresses bewilderment and disappointment). Is that happiness? What happiness is he talking about? Had Mobutu gone mad?
> [The performative moment:]
> Alex climbs down from the chair and steps closer to the audience as his voice becomes lower and softer. He smiles a real smile. In front of the

audience, as himself, he stretches out his hands and makes eye contact. Alex smiles a broad smile, it turns into a giggle and carries over to the audience. The audience responds in vocal cheers, laughter and a standing ovation that lasts for a minute or so.

In *IV Yes or IV No*, a performative moment takes place after the culminating scene in which Liat Haim buries Gushkale, her miscarried embryo. Iris, the performer, positions herself in a gynecological routine check-up position and Liat openly asks her doctor: 'Doctor, are you here because you really believe in what you're doing, or are you here to get rich off my illusions and everyone's expectations of me?' Liat stands up and declares: 'Doctor, I believe in my body in the simplest and clearest way.' It is then that the boundaries between Liat, the character, and Iris, the performer, blur as Iris turns directly to the audience in a performative moment:

> *So today I don't care if I were to have a boy or a girl*
> *If I were to become a mother*
> *Or would just stay an infertile woman...*

In three of the four performances, performatives took place during the performers' post-performance talks with the audience. Miki Peleg-Rothstein recalls that during such a talk in Tokyo, Japan, a woman in the uppermost balconies talked with great intensity for a long time. As she finished, the translator turned to Miki and dryly stated: 'it also happened to her.' Miki stood up and invited the woman to join her on stage. There they embraced and cried in each other's arms for several minutes (personal communication, 12/3/2014).

DISCUSSION

The performative in an autobiographical performance is a moment of transformation for both performer and audience occurring as a result of the dramatic action. Dramatically speaking, performatives are poignant moments of presence following climatic dramatic representations. In them the performer steps out of role to be present before the audience as themselves. Schechner (2009) depicts the state of presence as a '... falling out of character in so far as this character interferes with a direct communication of personality to the spectator' (p. 232).

In order for such moments to occur, performers engage in a preparatory process wherein they gradually reveal the essential aesthetic forms needed for the representation of their life stories. Reaching aesthetic distance in the preparatory process supports the performers in their personal processes, refines autobiographic representations and their communication to the audience and may be a necessary precursor to the experience of performatives in performance.

The director–performer alliance in DTAP corresponds to, and is based on, the therapeutic action in the creative arts therapies (Johnson, 1998). Externalization–transformation–internalization processes take place when the performer who has experienced trauma begins to internalize the role of survivor. The internalization process continues in performer–audience performatives and can eventually reach maturation. For instance, Maya Boltzmann recalls that the closing scene, where she stepped down from the table to reclaim Mirta, had changed and developed from one performance to the next. Through enactment, Maya's view of Mirta shifted progressively from a critical, shame-ridden and distanced stance to a sympathetic and loving reunion (personal communications, 12/17/2014).

CONCLUSION

In this chapter many similarities were revealed between APs and DTAPs. A three-phase structure consisting of preliminary, preparatory and performance phases was delineated and the fine balance existing between the reconstruction of representational forms and the spontaneous unfolding of performatives in autobiographical performances was examined. In addition, it was observed that performatives first occurred within the director–performer alliance and those were regarded as precursors to performatives in performance.

However, DTAPs differ from APs in regard to performatives on two counts. First, they seem to provide greater opportunity for performer–audience moments of meeting to take place. Second, the performer in DTAP is motivated to continue his/her performance only as long as it remains relevant to personal growth processes. Thus, Maya Boltzmann stopped performing *The Great Secret* soon after she was able express compassion towards her dead father and to fully reclaim Mirta into her adult life (personal communication, 12/17/2014). In other words, the double focus maintained in DTAPs makes them potentially more poignant and life-changing experiences, yet at the same time more transient than APs.

Further study is needed in examining the emergence of performative moments in APs and DTAPs, and their contribution to the theatrical and therapeutic processes within these two forms of performance of self. From this study, it appears that though the purpose of the two forms differ, the dynamics of performatives may be similar.

NOTE

1. Norman Issa, the director of 'Pshuta', was not interviewed for the study.

REFERENCES

Abramson, E. (2012). Instead of a child—After nine months a play was born (in Hebrew). *YNET*. Retrieved from http://www.ynet.co.il/articles/0,7340, L-4294770,00.html

Andersen, H. C. (1973). The snow queen. In *Andersen's fairy tales* (pp. 110–146). New York: Grosset & Dunlup Publishers.

Austin, J. L. (2007). How to do things with words: Lecture II. In H. Bial (Ed.), *The performance studies reader* (2nd ed., pp. 177–183). New York: Routledge.

Bailey, S. (2009). Performance in drama therapy. In D. R. Johnson & R. Emunah (Eds.), *Current approaches in drama therapy* (2nd ed., pp. 374–392). Springfield, IL: Charles C. Thomas Publishers.

Butler, J. (1988). Performative acts and gender constitution: An essay in phenomenology of feminist theory. *Theatre Journal, 40*(4), 519–531.

Butler, J. (1993). *Bodies that matter: On the discursive limits of 'Sex'*. New York: Routledge.

Dolan, J. (2005). *Utopia in performance: Finding hope at the theater*. Ann Arbor, MI: The University of Michigan Press.

Du Rand, L. (1992). Aesthetic and therapeutic inter-play in the creation of autobiographical theatre. *Arts in Psychotherapy, 19*, 209–218.

Emunah, R. (1994). *Acting for real: Drama therapy process, technique and performance*. New York: Brunner-Mazel.

Emunah, R. (2015). Self-revelatory performance: A form of drama therapy and theatre. *Drama Therapy Review, 1*(1), 71–85.

Fischer-Lichte, E. (2008). *The transformative power of performance: A new aesthetics*. New York: Routledge.

Foster, H. (1984). (Post)modern polemics. *New German Critique, 33*, 67–78.

Goffman, I. (1959). *The presentation of self in everyday life*. Garden City, NY: Doubleday.

Grotowski, J. (1986). *Towards a poor theatre*. London: Metheun.

Jacobson, R. (2006). Miki Peleg-Rothstein. *The British Theatre Guide*. Retrieved from http://www.britishtheatreguide.info/otherresources/interviews/Miki Peleg-Rothstein.htm

Johnson, D. R. (1998). On the therapeutic action of the creative arts therapies: The psychodynamic model. *Arts in Psychotherapy, 25*(2), 85–99.

Landy, R. (1986). *Drama therapy: Concepts and practices*. Springfield, IL: C. C. Thomas.

Lejeune, P. (1989). *On autobiography*. Minneapolis: University of Minnesota Press.

Rubin, T. (2010). Ladies' circle: A circle that touches pain (in Hebrew). *Ze Asher*. Retrieved from http://www.matteasher.org.il/info/docs/iton/asher61all.pdf

Schechner, R. (2009). *Performance theory*. New York: Routledge.

Snow, S., D'Amico, M., & Tanguay, D. (2003). Therapeutic theatre and well-being. *Arts in Psychotherapy, 30*, 73–82.

Stephenson, J. (2013). *Performing autobiography: Contemporary Canadian drama*. Toronto: University of Toronto Press.

Stern, D. N. (2004). *The present moment in psychotherapy and everyday life*. New York: W.W. Norton.

Thompson, J., & Schechner, R. (2004). Why 'social theatre'? *The Drama Review, 48*(3), 11–16.

Tronick, E. Z. (1998). Dyadically expanded states of consciousness and the process of therapeutic change. *Infant Mental Health Journal, 19*(3), 290–299.

Video Recordings of Performances

Boltzmann, M. (Producer and Performer), & Schnek-Yosef, O. (Director). (2009). *The Great Secret* [DVD in Hebrew]. Israel: Personal collection.

Harpaz, I. (Producer and Performer), & Schnek-Yosef, O. (Director). (2014). *IV Yes or IV NO: A Fertility Chart* [Video File in Hebrew]. Retrieved from https://www.youtube.com/watch?v=y6BvUqdZZow&list=UUkZrceZ05bvq bp6fNaF2N0A

Peleg-Rothstein, M. (Performer), & Issa, N. (Director). (2007). *Denuded* [DVD in Hebrew]. Israel: Habima, National Theatre Archives.

Vinegart, A. (Producer and Performer), & Shimshoni, L. (Director). (2012). *The Sad Tribe* [DVD in Hebrew]. Israel: The Israel Goor Theatre Archives and Museum at the Hebrew University of Jerusalem.

CHAPTER 12

Heuristic Methodology in Arts-Based Inquiry of Autobiographical Therapeutic Performance

Drew Bird

My intention is to present a framework for conducting arts-based inquiry into *autobiographical therapeutic performance* (ATP) as a performer, researcher and dramatherapist, based on Clark Moustakas' six phases of a heuristic methodology. The framework supports the centrality of performance and the theatrical art form in research in dramatherapy. The arts therapies professions often rely on the dominance of research approaches that use the written word; some 'do not yet see the links between artistic enquiry and formal research' (McNiff, 2013, p. 4). It is important that arts therapists do not lose their identity as artists. The dramatic art form can empower dramatherapists' practice as artists and subvert the dominance of the written word in research.

The framework combines solo performance and professional development using autobiographical material. It explores key themes including: the performer as artist and researcher; working with autobiographical and therapeutic material using metaphor; and the relationship between performer and audience. By exploring autobiographical material, one becomes more aware of how personal material impacts

D. Bird, MA, BSc.(Hons). PGCert. HE (✉)
College of Health and Social Care, University of Derby, Derby, UK
e-mail: D.P.Bird@derby.ac.uk

© The Author(s) 2016
S. Pendzik et al. (eds.), *The Self in Performance*,
DOI 10.1057/978-1-137-53593-1_12

169

the therapeutic relationship. This qualitative study, using ATP and theatre theory, will illustrate how performance can explore obstacles to forming intimate relationships and why play is important in this dynamic (Kumiega, 1987; Winnicott, 2005).

The framework proposed in this chapter synthesizes the roles of the artist, researcher and therapist, and resonates with *a/r/tography*—a research methodology that acknowledges one's role as an artist, researcher and teacher (Irwin, 2004). A/r/tography 'does not seek to answer questions or offer linear procedures that culminate in conclusions,' but is an ongoing process of active engagement and deeper understanding (Kalin, Lewis, & Steinecker, 2009, pp. 12–13). This is essentially a heuristic methodology.

Heuristic research is a qualitative research approach for understanding human experience and search for meaning, which is different from quantitative research, which is primarily concerned with measurement (Moustakas, 1994). The qualitative research view holds that knowledge is created from meaning and people's subjective interpretations of the social world (Matthews & Ross, 2010). Moustakas (1990), who uncovered the heuristic methodology, explores its Greek roots in the word 'heuriskein', which means to discover or find. The structure of the methodology resonates with the frame and container of a story used in dramatherapy that permits free, playful and creative exploration. Heuristic research helps to contain the chaotic processes of the artist, researcher and therapist, but is flexible enough to permit experimentation within the framework (Trimingham, 2002).

Heuristic research 'explicitly acknowledges the involvement of the researcher, to the extent that lived experience of the researcher becomes the main focus of the research' (Hiles, 2001, p. 3). The use of research participants helps to address the potential disequilibrium to 'help us avoid accusations of solipsism, self-indulgence, navel gazing or narcissism' (Etherington, 2004, p. 31). The involvement of participants, considered as co-researchers, helps to 'achieve richer, deeper, more profound, and more varied meanings' in the research process (Haertl, 2014; Moustakas, 1990, p. 47). The result is that the researchers' experience never stands alone (Etherington, 2004).

Moustakas (1990) suggests that heuristic research is about finding a question that needs illumination with a desire for understanding one's own experience. He identified the importance of entering into 'dialogue with the phenomenon' and 'being open and receptive to all aspects of one's experience' (p. 16). Arts-based enquiry can be used to dialogue with the senses and experiences of the body, and thus does not rely solely on verbal communication, but is open to body memories and other sensory modalities (Panhofer, Payne, Meekums, & Parke, 2011). Tacit knowing gives 'birth to the hunches and vague, formless insights that characterise heuristic discovery,' revealing hidden aspects of the self (Douglass & Moustakas, 1985, p. 49).

By using intuition, one draws on clues or patterns to bring greater understanding to one's experience. Curiosity drives the artist's endeavour: in the dramatic arts the performer wants to understand more fully a character's motivations, to get below the surface of superficial experience. Giving inner feelings, experiences and sensations an outward form helps to make one's experience more objective, and thus alleviate the potential dangers of being too inward-focused (Franklin, 2013). According to Moustakas (1990), focusing requires 'clearing an inward place' so one can tap into one's thoughts in a 'relaxed and receptive state' to achieve clarification (p. 25). By focusing on a physical sensation or a thought and examining one's experience, one goes beyond everyday experience (Douglass & Moustakas, 1985).

Etherington (2004) recognises how the research subject often has personal significance for the researcher, whether they are consciously or unconsciously aware of this. The internal frame of reference is informed by one's experience, 'one's perceptions, thoughts, feelings and sense' (Moustakas, 1990, p. 26). In this way one's awareness is not bound but open to the fullness of human experience and interpretation. In the framework of performance, the involvement of co-researchers (in the roles of director, supervisor and audience) helps to shed light on one's experience. This process resonates with the supervision process, whereby the supervisor is able to hold a mirror up to the therapist's experience to heighten awareness (Smith & Bird, 2014).

I believe that heuristic methodology is an excellent basis for an arts-based inquiry into ATP. The six phases of heuristic research identified by Moustakas (1990) will be applied to the methodology, artistic enquiry, autobiographical performance, personal and professional processes as a therapist. Moustakas' phases consist of: (1) initial engagement; (2) immersion; (3) incubation; (4) illumination; (5) explication; and (6) creative synthesis. It is important to recognise that heuristic research 'is not necessarily a linear process and certainly does not constitute a rigid framework', as one can move backwards or forwards at any time in the different phases (West, 2001, p. 129). The phases help to clarify the distinct features of heuristic research, but they should not be applied mechanistically. The phases show how the heuristic research frame has the potential to resonate with a therapeutic process and therapeutic theatre.

Case Example of an Autobiographical Therapeutic Performance

Applying Moustakas' six phases, I will now analyse one of my own ATP solo performance, using extracts from my personal journal. The performance is titled, *The god's play thing*, and portrays the myth of Psyche and Cupid in terms of absence and isolation. As the sole performer, I discover an empty stage and a cast that does not show up, and am forced to bring all my imaginary resources to bear to rescue the show from disaster. The show plays with the fine line between failure and success, and engages the audience in this effort. The first public performance was in November 2014 in Manchester, in a bare, medium-sized space in front of a small, intimate audience of ten people, consisting of creative arts therapists and friends.

Initial Engagement

Sela-Smith (2002) suggests that the subject of research needs to be a passionate concern, or something that calls out to the researcher with a sense of un-ease. Play helps to uncover passionate concerns that may reflect autobiographical material and unconscious experiences. Playing, devising and improvising can activate dormant experiences.

The performance began with the dramatic image of a man standing on an empty stage.

> *The image called out to me as having significant meaning. Isolation resonated as a passionate and existential concern that had potential autobiographic and therapeutic value. There was something about the challenge of being on an empty stage in front of an expectant audience that challenged me. There was certainly a degree of un-ease, perhaps even dis-ease. The un-ease is dramatized as I enter the stage, dismayed that the props and the cast are missing. Left to carry the story on my own I apologise to the audience, aware that some in the audience may find it tragic. Despite the challenging conditions and abandonment, I pledge to the audience I will carry the drama on my own.*

The sense of responsibility felt real and frightening. The image of Psyche being abandoned at the top of the mountain, tied to a tree and left to be devoured by a monster connected strongly with me at the initial stage of the research.

The heuristic approach resonates with arts-based research, requiring risk-taking, experimentation and discovery as well as 'a willingness… to tolerate chaotic or unpredictable states' (Kossak, 2013, p. 21). The approach encourages playing with one's fears, following one's instincts, suspending thought, and surrendering to impulses of the unknown (Sela-Smith, 2002). The notion of the artist as heuristic researcher keeps the tacit dimension active by sustaining a sense of mystery and the possibility of uncovering truths.

Immersion

This is where the researcher lives 'the question' daily, in both conscious and unconscious states; one is completely engaged in the process (Sela-Smith, 2002).

I wanted to explore the notion of isolation and abandonment. I have repeatedly had fearful dreams of being on stage in front of an audience and forgetting my lines. In the autobiographic drama I am left at the front of the church by a jilted lover as all the expectant guests look on. I rehearse and repeat the scene of abandonment again. The guests are all looking at me and they want answers. I flounder and try and find my voice. I am speechless and frozen. I am sweating. The theme of isolation appears again as I imagine myself as the abandoned Psyche tied to the tree. The image resonated with Christ on the cross and his final cry and torment of being abandoned by God. I immerse myself more fully in the scene, playing and replaying Psyche abandoned in the dark, cold and barren landscape.

Moments in the scene were intensified by focusing on specific actions, such as Psyche's shivers of excitement/fear, as she meets her fate. The cold hands, the chilblains and the scars from Psyche's hands were the paths I followed into the meaning of the piece.

The use of a dramatic metaphor lends itself to search and discovery; metaphors are not static, and their meanings can be reinterpreted many times. Immersing oneself deeply includes engaging the body, feelings and sensations, helping to elicit details from the devising process, and making it more real. The heuristic researcher strives to go beyond the limits of one's experience and knowledge, to extend awareness beyond the usual frontiers of knowing.

Incubation

Moustakas considered this phase a retreat from the phenomena in order for the 'inner tacit dimension to reach its full possibilities' (1990, p. 28). You cannot force discovery, but by retreating away from the intensity of the research or artistic endeavour the researcher is creating the conditions required for discovery (Djuraskovic & Arthur, 2010; Polyani, 1964).

In the devising process for ATP, the activation of the tacit dimension and the discovery of something new can happen inbetween rehearsals. Brook considered that 'it is important just to wait... (as)... coincidences and doors open by themselves' (1999, p. 114). By temporarily withdrawing, new dimensions of the devising experience open up without prompting.

I was aware that when I played Psyche, tied to the tree, I always looked left stage. I imagined she was looking for the monster and wasn't afraid. Then while drinking a cup of tea another meaning emerged: What if Psyche was avoiding looking at the audience? What if the audience was the monster and Psyche didn't want to face her fears? In the drama, Psyche was a willing sacrifice; she did not fear death. Yet there was a disparity between an idea for the drama and what I actually experienced physically in the dramatic moment. The realisation that the audience symbolically represented my fears proved to be a lynch pin in the final autobiographical performance.

Improvisation pushes against the boundaries of our everyday world, against the boundaries of our story, where we discover insight and thus create new works. The use of dramatic metaphor inherent in myth helps to turn the gaze away from the self and open up to the multiple interpretations permitted in the fictionalized realm. One is free to roam in an imaginary world beyond self-limiting beliefs, and remaining open to the unknown.

Illumination

Moustakas considers illumination as a breakthrough moment or an awakening that happens when one is 'open and receptive to tacit knowledge and intuition' (1990, p. 29). Acting first and thinking later keeps the tacit dimension alive. Staying with chaos within the playful state assures a living theatre, as opposed to a static theatre. Illumination in the devising process requires one to trust the process without forcing connections. Feedback from co-researchers amplifies many aspects of the performance. My director, Katy Tozer, also a dramatherapist, was able to bring both an artistic and therapeutic angle to the devising of my autobiographical performance. She commented on the sadness of one of the scenes involving a wedding. This feedback surprised me. I wanted to discover more about the scene and the dynamic with the expectant guests in their finery.

> *The groom is swallowed in silence. The audience wants an explanation. Where is the bride? The groom is frozen. He cannot move. Staying with the silence, the audience/wedding guests are all staring at me, recalling disappointment and unfulfilled expectation. Then the illumination—was this shame?*

The director was able to notice sadness in the scene, something that was outside of my immediate experience. The critical feedback from others helped to retain a measure of objectivity in the devising process.

I wanted to explore whether my autobiographical experiences had universal resonance for the audience. Following the show, some members of the audience were asked to provide feedback of their experience of the performance through email. Initially, I was concerned the audience would not share my experiences and I would feel alienated, but I had to take the risk of finding out whether the audience had connected with my performance.

> *One audience member commented about the intimacy created between the performer and audience, and on the bareness of the staging, which highlighted my vulnerability and thus facilitated her connection with the performance. I have often wondered whether I hide behind technique (such as using masks) in my practice as a dramatherapist. My instinct from the beginning was to have no props, lighting, costume nor stage scenery. I wanted to play with this un-ease that there was nowhere to hide. The audience member's feedback gave support to this risk I had taken.*

The illumination was a gradual awakening and realisation that I have a tendency to hide behind achievements or status that then become obstacles to intimacy. Perhaps I had doubted I was capable of the kind of intimacy required as a therapist. I felt exposed without stage scenery or props, but liberated and connected to the audience in an extraordinary way. I imagined

Clarkson's (2003) human to human connection, where therapist and client transcend the roles they play in the therapeutic dynamic.

By developing an awareness of one's habits and conditioning one is able to enter into a deeper and more meaningful relationship dynamic. In my performance, the empty space helped to dramatically intensify and illuminate my fears, raising my awareness and creating a new personal narrative (Bird, 2010).

Explication

The significant aspects of this phase are identifying major themes. By exploring specific moments in my autobiographical performance (e.g., focusing on a physical gesture or bodily sensation), themes that had therapeutic potential were magnified. Focusing in this way resonates with the work of Grotowski: digging deeper and deeper 'within an infinitely narrow band of experience' (Mitter, 1992, p. 133).

> I noticed Psyche had cord marks on her (my) wrists from her tied hands. Looking more closely at her freckled hands, her plain fingernails were clipped short and fine. She wanted her hands to look their finest for the monster. Details emerged as I noticed marks on her fingers where once were her precious rings. I was curious to discover that the rings had been removed by the crowd who escorted Psyche to the mountaintop, abandoning her to her fate. They had fought over her rings, especially the large emerald ring. As Psyche I share my bare and unadorned hands to the audience. The hands are ordinary, without pretense. The details of the marks left by the rings appeared at first as scars from an earlier life, then transformed into hands that could belong to a new story.

This explication process illuminated new themes, enabling me to reinterpret and question the scene in a different way. Due to the level of immersion in the process, I became aware of details that revealed information far beyond the outlines of the story, from other places and sources deep within the myth and my own personal past.

Creative Synthesis

Creative synthesis is the final phase that integrates meanings and themes helping to create an accurate depiction of experience (Moustakas, 1990). As I played out scenes and increased my physicality, details of memories emerged. The director offered ideas: 'Make it more physical, be more explicit, exaggerate the anxiety of being alone on stage and stay longer with feeling uncomfortable.'

I played with the idea of abandonment again, pacing backwards and forwards searching for the cast who had deserted the drama. I played with anxiety, awkwardness and embarrassment about being alone. There were long silences when I didn't know what to say or do. I wasn't used to everyone looking at me. Normally the audience looks at Psyche. It wasn't meant to be a one-man show. Eventually I had to confront the audience and face the responsibility I was struggling to own. I would have to tell the story of Psyche and Cupid on my own. No one was going to rescue me.

This moment was the first of many critical incidents that pointed to the notion of taking responsibility. It would be easy to blame the rest of the cast for abandoning me, but ultimately I needed to take ownership of the story. The feedback from the director brought my experience into dialogue, helped me to be more aware of my unease, and also validated my experience. We were not only co-researchers but co-creators. Through playful collaboration we were able to sustain the constant creative synthesis and re-visioning of theatrical ideas by heightening themes so they resonated more clearly (Heilpern, 1999). The sharing of an autobiographical performance helped me give up control of my experience and 'follow the surprise of what is emerging' (Levine, 2013, p. 21). The director's feedback helped encourage me to let go of one dramatic idea for the creation of another.

The synthesis raised my awareness of habits in my therapy practice, such as holding too tightly to a hypothesis about a client. The heuristic process offers a methodology to help one to keep exploring and to hold each discovery lightly until the next discovery unfolds. Moustakas recognised there was no endpoint in these explorations, seeing them as lifelong pursuits (Moustakas & Moustakas, 2004).

CONCLUSION

This chapter has explored the key concepts of heuristic research and illustrated how the six phases of the heuristic methodology are suited to an arts-based inquiry of autobiographical therapeutic performance. The importance of feedback from participants, directors, supervisor and audience to intensify the process of discovery has been emphasized, and demonstrated in excerpts from my own personal process in devising a performance. These phases are not rigid and should be used only as helpful guidelines in thinking about autobiographical therapeutic performance. Hopefully, this modest set of data can help to illuminate aspects of the self as artist, researcher and therapist.

REFERENCES

Bird, D. (2010). The power of a new story: The bigger picture. *Dramatherapy, 31,* 10–14.

Brook, P. (1999). *Threads of time: A memoir.* London: Methuen.

Clarkson, P. (2003). *The therapeutic relationship* (2nd ed.). London: Whurr.

Djuraskovic, I., & Arthur, N. (2010). Heuristic inquiry: A personal journey of acculturation and identity reconstruction. *Qualitative Report, 15,* 1569–1593.

Douglass, B. G., & Moustakas, C. (1985). Heuristic inquiry: The internal search to know. *Journal of Humanistic Psychology, 25,* 39–55.

Etherington, K. (2004). *Becoming a reflexive researcher—Using our selves in research.* London: Jessica Kingsley.

Franklin, M. A. (2013). Know thyself: Awakening self-referential awareness through art-based research. In S. McNiff (Ed.), *Art as research: Opportunities and challenges* (pp. 85–94). Chicago: Intellect.

Haertl, K. (2014). Writing and the development of the self-heuristic inquiry: A unique way of exploring the power of the written word. *Journal of Poetry Therapy, 27,* 55–68.

Heilpern, J. (1999). *Conference of the birds: The story of Peter Brook in Africa.* London: Routledge.

Hiles, D. (2001). *Heuristic inquiry and transpersonal research.* In CCPE Conference, London, UK. October 2001. Accessed August 26, 2015, from http://psy.dmu.ac.uk/drhiles/HIpaper.htm

Irwin, R. L. (2004). A/r/tography: A metonymic metissage. In R. L. Irwin & A. de Cosson (Eds.), *A/r/tography: Rendering self through arts based living inquiry* (pp. 27–40). Vancouver, BC: Pacific Educational Press.

Kalin, N., Lewis, L., & Steinecker, D. (2009). *Exploring the landscapes or arts based educational research.* Paper presented at the National Art Educational Association Annual Convention (Research Division), Minneapolis, MN.

Kossak, M. (2013). Art-based enquiry: It is what we do! In S. McNiff (Ed.), *Art as research: Opportunities and challenges* (pp. 19–27). Chicago: Intellect.

Kumiega, J. (1987). *The theatre of Grotowski.* London: Methuen.

Levine, S. (2013). Expecting the unexpected: Improvisation in art-based research. In S. McNiff (Ed.), *Art as research: Opportunities and challenges* (pp. 125–132). Chicago: Intellect.

Matthews, B., & Ross, L. (2010). *Research methods: A practical guide for the social sciences*. Harlow, UK: Pearson Education Ltd.

McNiff, S. (2013). Opportunities and challenges in art based research. In S. McNiff (Ed.), *Art as research: Opportunities and challenges* (pp. 3–9). Chicago: Intellect.

Mitter, S. (1992). *Systems of rehearsal: Stanislavsky, Brecht, Grotowski, and Brook*. London: Routledge.

Moustakas, C. (1990). *Heuristic research: Design, methodology, and applications*. London: Sage.

Moustakas, C. (1994). *Phenomenological research methods*. Thousand Oaks, CA & London: Sage.

Moustakas, C. E., & Moustakas, K. (2004). *Loneliness, creativity and love: Awakening meaning in life*. New York: Xlibris.

Panhofer, H., Payne, H., Meekums, B., & Parke, T. (2011). Dancing, moving and writing in clinical supervision? Employing embodied practices in psychotherapy supervision. *Arts in Psychotherapy, 38,* 9–16.

Polyani, M. (1964). *Science, faith and society*. Chicago: University of Chicago Press.

Sela-Smith, S. (2002). Heuristic research: A review and critique of Moustakas' method. *Journal of Humanistic Psychology, 42,* 53–88.

Smith, M. E., & Bird, D. (2014). Fairy tales, landscapes and metaphor in supervision: An exploratory study. *Counseling and Psychotherapy Research: Linking Research with Practice, 14,* 2–9.

Trimingham, M. (2002). A methodology for practice as research. *Studies in Theatre and Performance, 22,* 54–60.

West, W. (2001). Beyond grounded research: The use of a heuristic approach to qualitative research. *Counseling and Psychotherapy Research, 1,* 126–131.

Winnicott, D. W. (2005). *Playing and reality*. London: Routledge.

CHAPTER 13

A Retrospective Study of Autobiographical Performance During Dramatherapy Training

Ditty Dokter and Alida Gersie

HISTORY OF AUTOBIOGRAPHICAL PERFORMANCE IN BRITISH DRAMATHERAPY TRAINING PROGRAMS

Since 1986 three British dramatherapy training programs have required trainees to develop and present their own autobiographical performance to audiences of peers, other university students, staff, clinical supervisors and guests. After discussing the origins of the pedagogical decision to require this, we outline our research into the memories of practicing dramatherapists about these performances—some of which took place over twenty years ago. Included are the dramatherapists' own words for their experiences. We highlight the relevance of our findings for current dramatherapy practice and research.

In the mid-1980s dramatherapy tutors at Hertfordshire College of Art & Design (hereafter the St Albans/Hatfield course) pioneered the trainees' creation and showing of an autobiographical performance. At present, all UK Masters in Dramatherapy include student-created performance(s) in their teaching and learning strategies. Two of these training programs

D. Dokter, PhD (✉)
Anglia Ruskin University, Cambridge, UK
e-mail: dittydokter@googlemail.com

A. Gersie, PhD
Independent Researcher and Organization Consultant, London, UK
e-mail: alidasg@icloud.com

require an explicit autobiographic focus. Below we discuss the rationale behind the inclusion of such 'theatre of the self' in UK dramatherapy training. Following an outline of research methods we thematically analyze the written and oral memories of these performances by 15 practicing dramatherapists. We then highlight some implications of our findings for contemporary dramatherapy practice.

During its early years, the part-time dramatherapy course in St. Albans/Hatfield (1977–1983) engaged trainees with clinical theory and practice, drama/theatre processes, a dramatherapy training group, and individual and group performances around generic themes. These performances were shown to an intimate audience of fellow students and tutors. In 1982, the course failed its first application to the Council for National Academic Awards (CNAA) for provisional validation at postgraduate level, which was a severe blow. It prevented, for example, state funding for course delivery, deprived trainees of grants for their studies and put a halt to the development of pay scales for dramatherapists in the NHS, Social Services and Education. The absence of a dramatherapy-based pedagogic rationale for the performances had confirmed the CNAA's panel's impression that dramatherapy was simply a newfangled name for already well-established practices in recreational drama, drama-in-education, community drama and psychodrama. They also noted that the performances failed to take account of recent developments in experimental and community theatre.

At the time these performances had taken a strong monologic and political turn. Plays and workshops by Dario Fo and Franca Rame, for example, unleashed fierce debate about theatre's role in examining the links between identity, oppression and liberation. Self-exploratory approaches to performance in feminist, black, disability and community theatre addressed kindred themes. This heady mix of innovatory theatre methods challenged traditional understandings of the relationships between performer, play, context and spectator. In new and established performance spaces alike, the audience's experience of culturally construed identities and their entailed social constrictions or prohibitions was dramatically deconstructed, explored and re-formed (van Erven, 1988). The shows reflected their makers' budding awareness of the dynamics of intersubjectivity that informed the discourses and indeed the practices of artists, psychotherapists, teachers and social workers alike (Stern, 2004).

Before long newly appointed tutors redesigned the curriculum of the St Albans/Hatfield course. Informed clinical thinking and the supervision of clinical practice became central to training. The content of drama/theatre courses was restructured along developmental lines, while dramatherapy theory became rooted in attachment theory (Bowlby, 1969), developmental approaches (Johnson, 1982), symbolic interaction (Rose, 1962), narrative psychology (Sarbin, 1986) and social constructionism (Bannister, 1977). Broadly interactionist ideas, such as agency, communication, meaning-making, symbolization and emergence, were dramatically explored (see also Brisset & Edgley, 1974). Artistic skill (Bateson, 1970) combines many levels of mind, not a single level.

In 1985–86 the decision was made to require trainees to create autobiographical performances of 25–30 minutes' duration. Tutors thought that the making and showing of these 'theatres of selves-in-relation' would help trainees to embody their learning on the course. It would engage them with key dramatherapeutic concerns, such as how to facilitate the development of more productive connections between self, others and society; and how to engage constructively with diversity issues, intimacy, exigencies of time and place, and meaning-making. The very doing of the autobiographical performances would also raise therapeutically important ethical topics, such as respect for the uniqueness of the other, privacy, confidentiality and its limits, misdirected or covert self-revelation and intentional secret-keeping. Thanks to this extensive redesign, the St Albans/Hatfield course achieved provisional validation by the CNAA in 1986 and final validation in 1989. Soon after, the professional title *Dramatherapist* was protected by law in the UK. Anyone using the title must be registered with the Health and Care Professions Council.

The decision to include autobiographical performances (AP) in dramatherapy training was timely and prescient. Since then general interest in autobiography has burgeoned as expressed in books, public performances and in the *dramatisation-of-self* via social media and networking. Performance artists continue to use personal experience as vehicles through which to project distinct social perspectives inflected by positions of race, class, gender and/or sexuality. Their shows protest against marginalisation and objectification. They aim to reveal invisible lives and to facilitate self-agency (Govan, Nicholson, & Normington, 2007; Heddon, 2008). The work of many performance artists and autobiographical actors can be considered as an act of recovery achieved through the empowering effect of constructing a narrative around traumatic experiences (Heddon, 2008, p. 54). Baker's show, *Portraits of Living with Mental Illness* (2010), parallels the work of *I can't believe we're not better* (www.charitychoice, 2014) and Drama Lab NYC (Sajnani, 2012) by drawing attention to the relationship between agency and mental health. The concept of identity as performatively constructed (Butler, 1997) is nowadays integral to dramatherapy training and practice. Countless autobiographical performances are designed and performed within the privacy of ongoing dramatherapy groups. Several advocacy theatre companies such as *I can't believe we're not better* have been initiated from such clinical practice, in this case by the dramatherapist Gerald Maiello (www.Ican'tbelievewe'renotbetter.co.)

The distinctions between the terms *self-revelatory performance, autobiographical and therapeutic theatre* have recently been delineated by Renée Emunah (2015), though until now they have been used interchangeably in the UK. Historically, the effects of one-time and repeated APs have been discussed by Emunah and Johnson (1983) and Pendzik (1988). Their writings consider the importance of ensemble and internal/external connections to both the content of the play and with a semi-public or public audience (Emunah & Johnson, 1983) and the therapeutic development of an autobiographical play and its presentation in front of an audience (Pendzik, 1988). In Europe the curative effectiveness of in-group as well as public performance were highlighted (Bailey, 2009; Yotis, 2002). Jacques (2011) has more recently described the impact of repetition and public performance on clients with regard to agency development and user involvement in the treatment and service delivery for mental illness.

In her seminal article Emunah (2015) distinguishes between autobiographical and self-revelatory theatre as follows:

> Self-revelatory performance (hereafter referred to as Self-Rev) is similar to autobiographical theatre, but with two clear distinctions. In Self-Rev there is an unambiguous attempt at 'working through' the presented material. Autobiographical theatre (Heddon, 2008), on the other hand, involves dramatic storytelling or dramatization of personal life material, but without a conscious aim of healing or transforming this material. The performer focuses on current issues or dilemmas, whereas autobiographical theatre most often revolves around stories or experiences from the past. Self-Rev issues may well stem from the past, and pertain to ongoing life themes, but the focus is on how these issues impact the performer's present life'. (p. 72)

In another recent publication, Sajnani (2012) emphasizes relational aesthetics, arguing the importance of the audience's presence as witness, but also the importance of relationship in witnessing in order not to 'eroticise injury' (p. 7). There are, Sajnani says, 'tremendous opportunities for radical intimacy, healing and social change for performers and audience, when these relationships are made visible and available to public interaction' (p. 8).

METHODOLOGY

We wondered what graduates might remember about their autobiographical performances during training, and if/how there were resonances between their memories and the pedagogic rationale for the APs in training. We used diverse data sources common to qualitative research (Bryman, 2012) to explore our query. These are:

1. Archival data such as course documents and student handbooks.
2. Semi-structured questionnaires.
3. In-depth individual interviews.
4. Content analysis with independent topic identification and rating.

Respondents

Eighteen people responded to our call for Participation in Research made to members of the British Association of Dramatherapists in August 2014. All received a detailed research description; 15 returned the completed questionnaire and ten were interviewed. All respondents were volunteer graduates of the three institutions that included autobiographical performance(s) during training. The respondents included 12 women and three men. Six respondents graduated between 1989 and 1999; three between 2000 and 2008, and seven between 2009 and 2014 from the University of Hertfordshire (previously the St Albans/Hatfield course), Roehampton University and Anglia Ruskin University. The interviews followed the format of the questionnaire. The interviews were transcribed and checked for accuracy with the interviewees.

Memory-Evoking Queries

We formulated memory-evoking queries in the following domains:

1. The creation and doing of the AP during training, such as title, the selection of a focus or foci; dramatic forms considered and used;

self-revelation; the roles of tutors, peers, partner, friends and/or family during the process.

2. Audience: such as audience–composition and responses.
3. Any persistence of memories of the AP post-training; the possible emergence of further meanings; and potential effects on his/her work as a dramatherapist.
4. Any other comments.

Content Analysis

In analyzing the transcripts of the interviews, we identified five main themes: dramatic forms; relationships; privacy; participation/collaboration/witnessing; and diversity. In our analysis we stayed aware of the normal complexities of qualitative research such as the (un)reliability of evoked memories of historical events, the bias generated by the prescribed focus of questionnaires and interviews and the inevitable influence of interviewer/interviewee dynamics on what respondents write or say (Giele & Elder, 1998).

Dramatic Forms

All respondents knew when starting their training that they were required to do an AP. Several remembered feeling very excited by this and by the thought that they could use dramatic media, styles and expressive forms that suited the focus of their piece and stretched their creative ability. Referring to his AP of nearly two decades previously, Kevin wrote: 'I recall pushing out the boat as it were. I used movement, mime, puppetry, mask-work, sound, dance, music and sculpts to help create different terrains, landscapes, people and dwelling places.' The AP was, he recalled, steeped in metaphor. Kevin reminded us that he was born in Britain but of Jamaican descent. The fact that his brother, whose terminal illness was the focus of this AP, was born in Jamaica but raised in the UK had made him decide to set his AP in 'a mystical country, unknown and abroad'. He represented England as 'another unique place—beyond space and time'. He remembered that he cast several co-students as his brother, his brother's closest friends and lovers, and his own alter-ego. He played himself as a 'character who might have looked like an African prince'. The script was a reality-based, descriptive story, which he narrated and pre-recorded. All acting, including his own, was performed silently, using diverse miming techniques and movement. He recalled using the 'as if' by changing all names to African names. Though the actual events represented in both story and play took place between 1985 and 1995, he replaced what could have been modern dress with timeless Egyptian style robes and full face masks.

Five other respondents whose APs were, like Kevin's, reality-oriented but infused with the imaginary, similarly chose a rich combination of dramatic forms. They did so, they recalled, because the mix enabled them to use both direct self-revelation and metaphoric representation of their issues and experiences. Bianca, for example, had wanted to use her AP to present a process of learning to face her fear of anger and change her tendency to project anger onto others. The AP was based on the story of Little Red Riding Hood. At one point she remembers voicing the grandmother's fear of the wolf as an exterior threat: 'He's out there, roaming, seeking, lurking.' Later she had been able to say quite firmly in the role of the grandmother: 'He's my wolf then. He's not out there. He belongs to me.' This statement, Bianca reflected, was an overt revelation of her struggle with anger. She had found it personally and professionally helpful that this revelation was contained by the role and the story.

Five others used an entirely metaphorical structure. Seven years post-qualifying, Nick described his AP as a non-verbal piece with movement, voice, music and mime in which he used the metaphor of a matador at a bullfight. Within the 'revealing privacy' of this metaphor, Nick remained fully aware of what each scene represented for him—the call to train as a dramatherapist, feeling intimidated by academic requirements, experiences of involuntary childlessness, Christian faith, the impact of studying part-time, and his passion for theatrical processes and witnessing. He did not know if his audience grasped these links, but this did not matter to him. Tina also worked entirely metaphorically. In addition to using mime, movement and music, she remembered creating paintings on canvas, blowing up balloons and using a red cape to represent her feelings of loss, isolation and fear. She vividly remembered using this red cape at a late point in her AP to create the shape of a baby. Though she rehearsed this symbolic transformation many times, during her actual performance she suddenly realized that the red cape represented a younger version of herself. This realization was accompanied by an overwhelming sense that she needed to nurture her inner child. Its undeniable clarity helpfully guided her healing pathway in subsequent years.

A further five respondents created explicit, episodic montages of autobiographical memories. In addition to scripted text, these APs involved photographs, fragments from diaries and other writings, tableaux-vivants, enacted scenes, snippets of film and audio recordings. Some included childhood toys, familiar objects or relatives' clothes. These respondents emphasized that they had grasped the opportunity to create an explicit AP. Deborah, for example, knew from the beginning that she would use her AP to rework painful memories from her childhood in Northern Ireland during the 'Troubles'. These memories included hearing the sirens of fire engines and ambulances, witnessing bomb explosions, and seeing helicopters flying overhead. She dramatized her young presence near burning vehicles, men with guns and masks, fighting, conflict with the police, family death and conflicts over flags. Doing the AP, Deborah said, gave her a much better understanding of what the events and the omnipresent shadow of the conflict meant to her. She wanted her audience to understand that parts of her were 'lost and shattered into pieces because of the Troubles'. She hoped that the performance might help her to begin to gather herself again, as indeed it did. She wanted the causes of her shattering to be explicit and therefore used, she said, unambiguous representations of the 'Troubles' in the form of photos, video clips, descriptive and poetic texts as well as sounds.

Relationships Unveiled

Ten respondents remembered using their AP to clarify a pattern of family relationships or disturbing external events. In her AP, Gaby made visible 'for the first time' the complex dynamics of growing up in one of her childhood homes, though she felt: 'Oh my God, am I being disloyal?' Like other respondents, she felt little 'inner choice' about the relational focus of her AP. 'I cannot say exactly why I chose her (mother) as the main theme. I think the theme chose me at that moment, something wanted to be publicly made visible, shown and witnessed' (Gaby). Kevin felt the same undeniable pull. He 'had to explore' his warring and loving relationship with his eldest blood brother, the brother's discovery of his sexuality and the brother's terminal illness around the time of the AP. During a preparatory workshop, when Ida felt 'utterly undecided' about the focus of her AP she experienced a wave of flashback memories related to her older brother, which settled her AP's focus. Throughout their childhood her brother experienced severe behavioral difficulties. During adolescence he became violent towards their parents. Though this was very frightening and unsettling for Ida and her younger sister, the girls' fear and sadness about what was going on at home were not heard in the family or elsewhere. When she was 13, Ida described the menacing events at home in an essay for her religious education tutor. She did so 'in order to be heard, but nobody picked it up'. Ida developed her AP about 12 years after the submission of that essay. At the time her brother's behavior was still difficult, though no longer violent. What matters here is that 16 years after her AP, and therefore about 28 years after the deeply disturbing period, Ida, who currently works in an adult mental health setting, joined our research in order to underline just how important having those experiences witnessed, empathized with and understood remained to her. She wanted to make it unambiguously clear that the AP and the audience responses had helped her to begin to own feelings such as sadness and fear which she had until then brushed aside.

Five trainees in our sample primarily used their AP to examine, display and improve their relationship with an aspect of themselves that they felt hampered by: a tendency to withdraw from social contact when things became tough; a fear of anger; a habit of creating chaos (literally and metaphorically) in their immediate, physical surroundings. The opportunity provided by the AP to reveal and surmount these dynamics, mostly through metaphor, was likewise experienced as 'immensely helpful'. A majority of respondents stated that 'having been embedded in personal therapy' (a training requirement) had given psychological support for the intense AP process. It also enabled the working through of material that could not be processed in the learning environment of the training context.

Layers of Privacy
Several respondents shared that though their AP's content might have seemed explicitly self-disclosing, their self-revelation was actually deeply layered, with some layers being kept deliberately hidden from the audience. At the time of performance all were aware that elements of their AP would mean different things to different people depending on the depth and quality of their relationship with them. As such, every AP functioned somewhat like a Johari window, a tool to help people better understand their relationship with self and others (Luft & Ingham, 1955). It clarified whether the AP content was already known to oneself or known to others. All respondents noted that they knowingly chose comfortable levels of concealment and revelation in their AP. Several respondents said that they encoded important hidden information in the music that they played or sung during their AP but had not divulged the music's significance

while performing. Cecily explained that among her invitees some would have immediately understood a certain sung reference in her AP. Others would not, though she hoped that some of those might have guessed its meaning. She revealed that five years post-performance there was still one element of her AP that she had not yet explained to anyone (nor did she want to speak explicitly about this at the time of the interview).

Two respondents shared that they learned from immediate post-performance feedback that their AP had unveiled aspects of their life experience to members of the audience which had until then been unacknowledged by themselves. When they received this feedback both felt that the audience's perception connected deeply to their lived reality. They were then able to work on the issues raised in a healing way.

Respondents stressed the importance of the performer's need to feel comfortable with the anticipated consequences, the chosen mode of performance, and the context in which the self-revelation happens. Most respondents remembered being deeply aware that their disclosure would affect the quality of their future relations with individual members of their diverse audience. Indeed it was the goal of the AP to make this happen. Ultimately, however, such consequences are unpredictable. Respondents were glad to have taken time to foresee with some accuracy any consequences that could be predicted.

Participation, Collaboration and Witnessing

While some respondents remembered their AP as very much a solo process, most involved peers in the different stages of devising, rehearsing and performing. Doing so raised several issues, which were clearly articulated by Leon. He commented that:

> 'The input from peers was hugely varied. By this point in the training there were fellow students whose opinions I trusted implicitly and I welcomed their input and reflections. Again, this influenced my final performance in the same manner as the tutor's reflections. For others, I listened to what they had to say, but recognized that I had to be truthful to my intent behind the performance. During rehearsals some had relied heavily on their peers as mirrors who gave useful feedback. Others noted that because they were required to be their own playwright, lead actor, director and producer, they gladly delegated the other roles of a theatre company, such as stagehands, stage manager, light and sound operator, to one or more of their peers. Some also used peers as actors or were actors in their peers' APs.

The reciprocal collaboration was reflected in comments such as: 'My fellow students were wonderfully supportive, and came to all the rehearsals' (Kevin); and 'I'm not sure I've ever felt such support in my life before or since' (Esther).

Fiona was asked to play someone's grandmother and to speak in this woman's mother tongue, a language she did not speak. She had found this responsibility 'more nerve wracking than doing her own'. Ida also happily remembered, 'having a role in a funeral scene' in a peer's AP as well as technical responsibilities in another. Having been able to perform these collaborative tasks remained very important to several of our respondents.

Some respondents remembered deciding early on that they would work mostly alone. Gaby noted that she works best in isolation. Nick stated that he did not feel the need to include anyone else in either his rehearsal or his performance process: 'I was probably feeling very vulnerable and used the option of staying alone through the creative process as a way of protecting myself.' He simply asked a friend for some music he wanted to use, and showed his partner some of the work; he would have felt hampered 'with someone else giving their opinions'. He felt confident enough, he added, 'to risk working completely alone'.

Trainees without an active role in another trainee's performance were expected to join the general audience and become a witness to that performance. Gaby described this as 'an expectation to hold the space for the self-revelatory process to unfold, and to be an audience in the theatrical sense of providing an essential dynamic in the performance-process that occurs between actor, the dramatic narrative and those watching it' (see also Emunah, Raucher, & Ramirez, 2014; Emunah, 2015). We found it interesting that many respondents spontaneously noted that, 'being understood by their audience had not been of prime importance to them.' Alyssa wrote: 'I'm not sure if the wider audience understood the meaning of my self-revelation in the parts of the performance where I shared in a more metaphorical way. It did not matter as I imagine the tone and more universal symbols were clear and may have resonated for individuals.'

Bianca was not sure either if the wider audience had understood the meaning of her self-revelation. She said: 'Often the dynamic between actor and audience can enliven or deaden a performance. I sensed intuitively that they were engaged and this is what mattered. The dynamism created an energy between us that allowed the performance to happen.' Though unsure about the audience's understanding of the meaning of his performance, Kevin felt certain about the audience's connection with him and his fellow actors during his performance. 'I felt an electricity in the air when we started performing... they were really enthralled... there was a lot of cheering afterwards and I recall sitting in a huge circle... sharing feedback.'

In all trainings the APs were shown to an invited audience in quick succession. Fiona said that as a performer there had only been 'a bit of time' to absorb the audience's responses. Several respondents mentioned that they had found this switch in attention from their own AP to collaborating with or watching others very helpful. Many respondents commented on the profound sense of camaraderie with their fellow students, the buzz around preparing the work as well as the excitement of seeing the performances. The intense, emotional arousal of the APs seems to affect the long-term recall of their impact. To this day Hanna vividly remembers the visual image of the Cross on the ground in her AP, the silence in the room, the African spiritual song she sang, the poem that a fellow student who was a good friend wrote and read for her, as well as the emotion and catharsis, which she defined as release, that she felt after the performance.

Here three features strike us. First, most respondents clearly remembered many years later that their AP involved other people. Secondly this co-presence mattered greatly, both at the time and in hindsight. This finding suggests that the participative, joint effort and solidarity characteristics of the entire AP process deserve to be closely examined. In this context it is also worth noting Nick's comment that he might have been too vulnerable to share the creation of his performance with others.

Diversity

Our respondents identified diversity-related issues such as disability, ethnicity, nationality, religion, class and age as being important to their explorations. Two participants self-identified as black, the others as white. Three were male; 13 female. All used English as their mother tongue. Two respondents now practice overseas. While some respondents, like Kevin, Cynthia and Martha, used their AP to explore issues of diversity related to sexual orientation, ethnic or racial background and/or disability, others held back from doing so. The decision to engage with contentious topics depended in part, according to Nick, on earlier peer responses. At some point, he said, a fellow student had been almost vitriolic about Christians. Being the only man in a large group of female students he had thought: 'I already have enough problems and pressures. Being a Christian is not easy' and he did not want to make things worse for himself. As he presented his AP at the end of training it felt safe to clearly identify himself as a Christian. In her AP, Hannah explored her experience of crossroads related to her

Christian background as well as a more general sense of displacement. It was helpful, she said, that some peers shared her displacement, though overall there remained a sense of isolation for her. She said: 'Outwardly I showed anger. Inwardly I felt loss and separation. I interpreted my classmates... not understanding me, as based on my internal working model at the time.' Anger at being/having been misunderstood often arises when diversity becomes a theme for the AP. One respondent who was diagnosed with dyslexia during training said: 'Right up to when I came to train and whilst I was training too, I suppose my behavior was at times irrational. At times I was angry. There was a period I lost a sense of who I was. I think it was OK, but when I heard some concerns from family and friends it made me stop and think. Going through the AP process helped me understand the way my younger self had behaved.'

Those performers who were survivors of the harmful effects of prejudice and/or experienced the AP process as both a significant challenge and an extraordinary opportunity. Kevin said that because some diversity issues were simultaneously addressed in lectures and workshops, it made it easier for him to make sense of what he had experienced.

APs as Personal Development in Dramatherapy Training

Most respondents commented that they could not really imagine doing a dramatherapy training that did not include an AP. When asked why, Nick explained that: 'doing the AP is about owning—as therapists—our drama that goes on inside us'. From his perspective our experiences get locked in our bodies. When released through the AP, 'this does something spiritual to both performer and their audience'. Ida stated, 'It was cathartic. I think it was extremely helpful for me to deal with some of my experiences and feelings that I had brushed aside and being able to reflect on them, their impact on me as a therapist and taking them to therapy. I would say it was a very therapeutic experience for me. I include performing in other students' performances in that. It was also helpful in understanding experientially the power of theatre, the therapeutic potential, and the need for boundaries and rituals.'

Irrespective of how long ago they did their AP, all respondents emphasized that they continued to this day to work with the themes, dynamics and emotions of the AP. Bianca said: 'It has had a far-reaching effect on my life. With a significant dream, Jung believed it was important not to analyse it too soon, but to circumambulate it and allow the meanings to emerge' (Stevens, 1990, p. 107). 'This walking around the experience of my autobiographical performance has not been continual for me but rather a form of re-visiting the memory every now and then and seeing what I find. I chose to work with an archetypal story, which holds pro-found meaning for me in terms of facing fear, transforming anger and gaining new perspectives. The symbols within it are still working actively in my life.' Nick said seven years later: 'It is still as alive in me today as when I first performed it... I regard it a bit like a spring of fresh water that revives and replenishes. The title is certainly something that continues to show me what lies beneath, psychically hidden and coming into the fore-front of my mind when needed.'

When these respondents mindfully revisit their AP they develop, in their terms, some kind of new perspective on their lives. The memory constitutes embodied awareness of the dynamics of change, which, in turn, affects their practice as dramatherapists. Olga said that her AP expe-rience strengthened her passion for and belief in the impact of creative engagement on people. It had 'contributed to relationships both person-ally and professionally'. Ida's experience helps her to ensure to this day that she uses personal experiences safely in therapy and to see 'when and why she may have strong transference responses' to certain aspects of clients' lives. For Cecily, the AP served to increase her respect for what it takes to face fears and a secure knowledge that personal transforma-tion is possible. Nearly twenty years after his AP, Kevin observed that 'the biography' continues to inform his view that 'everyone—no matter how shy or unconfident or disabled you are—everyone has a story to tell and that can be through movement, drama, art, music, dance or words'. Alyssa, a more recent graduate, spoke for many others in her comment that: 'In terms of understanding myself, my potential in becoming a dramatherapist and understanding my potential client's experience, the APs were invaluable.'

Points raised about potentially problematic areas included consider-ations of timing of the performance within the training, the nature of the audience and the type and focus of assessment. Participants also pointed out that their thoughts and feelings about these problematic areas had been subject to significant reassessment over time. All respondents felt that the process of doing APs increased their efficacy in helping clients to surmount their intrapsychic and interpersonal difficulties.

CONCLUSION

This chapter addressed the specific short- and long-term memories of APs created by practicing dramatherapists, in the course of their study for a UK postgraduate degree in dramatherapy. The freshness of their memories was startling. Older memories can be reported from a distant point of view. In our research this rarely happened. Most of the time respondents spoke or wrote about their AP as if it happened recently.

Autobiographical memories encompass wide-ranging knowledge, insights, facts and intuitions; they are a gorgeous miscellany of semantic details and episodes. We found that the memories evoked by our research were similarly extensive. They served a wide range of adaptive, social, directive-giving and self-representational functions for each individual.

Our participants produced a rich variety of responses. The core theme analysis of the 16 descriptive questionnaires and ten in-depth interviews, which we have presented, identified some important characteristics of doing APs during dramatherapy training, which merit further research:

- When to develop selected intrapsychic and/or interpersonal relationships into a dramatic performance (and when not);
- The benefits and risks of reciprocal collaboration with fellow group-members as actors, stagehands/technicians and audience/witnesses;
- The therapeutic benefits of learning to deal with 'layered privacy' in and beyond the AP;
- The embodiment of aesthetic distance by juggling metaphoric and direct self-revelation;
- Awareness that others/audiences subjectively interpret what they witness and will consequently take from a situation/performance what they want;
- The realization that memories and life experiences are co-constructed and re-constructed, and the role of culture in this process;
- Making connections between the AP and the skills at clinical practice.

Our respondents reported that doing their AP had resulted in enduring and productive personal change. The changes were manifest in relationships with self, peers, friends and/or family, and had been recognized as such by these important others. Their memories of the APs suggest that the original pedagogic rationale for introducing autobiographical performances in dramatherapy training has stood the test of time.

Acknowledgements We would like to thank those who would rather not be named (pseudonyms have been used throughout this chapter), as well as Eva Marie Bryer, Michelle Buckley, Terence Clay, Peter Darby Knight, Christian Dixon, Clare Hubbard, Annabel Maidment, Ciara McClelland, Emma Ramsden, Bea Scott, and Jessica Williams-Ciemnyjewski for their contributions to this research.

References

Bailey, S. (2009). Performance in drama therapy. In D. R. Johnson & R. Emunah (Eds.), *Current approaches in drama therapy* (pp. 374–389). Springfield, IL: Charles C. Thomas.

Baker, B. (2010). *Portraits of mental illness.* Accessed January 23, 2015, from www. theguardian.com/artanddesign/video/2010/may/12/art-mental-illness

Bannister, D. (Ed.) (1977). *New perspectives in personal construct theory.* London: Academic Press.

Bateson, G. (1970). *Form, substance and difference.* Nineteenth Annual Korzybski Lecture, delivered January 9, 1970, under the Auspices of the Institute of General Semantics. General Semantics Bulletin, No. 37.

Bowlby, J. (1969). *Attachment. Attachment and loss* (Vol. *1*). New York: Basic Books.

Brisset, D., & Edgley, C. (Eds.) (1974). *Life as theatre: A dramaturgical source-book.* Chicago: Transaction Publishers.

Butler, J. (1997). *Excitable speech: A politics of the performative.* London: Routledge.

Bryman, A. (2012). *Social research methods.* Oxford: Oxford University Press.

Calle, S. (2007). *Take care of yourself.* https://www.youtube.com/watch?v=cRx7nFVuLwA

Emunah, R. (2015). Self-revelatory performance: A form of drama therapy and theatre. *Drama Therapy Review, 1,* 71–85.

Emunah, R., & Johnson, D. R. (1983). The impact of theatrical performance on the self-image of psychiatric patients. *Arts in Psychotherapy, 10,* 233–239.

Emunah, R., Raucher, G., & Ramirez, A. (2014). Self-revelatory performance in mitigating the impact of trauma. In N. Sajnani & D. Johnson (Eds.), *Trauma-informed drama therapy* (pp. 93–121). Springfield, IL: Charles C. Thomas.

Giele, J. Z., & Elder, G. H. (1998). *Methods of life-course research.* London: Sage.

Govan, E., Nicholson, H., & Normington, K. (2007). *Making a performance: Devising histories and contemporary practices.* London: Routledge.

Heddon, D. (2008). *Autobiography and performance.* London: Palgrave Macmillan.

'I can't believe I'm not better' theatre company (2014). Accessed December 6, 2014, from www.charitychoice.icantbelievewerenotbetter.org

Jacques, J.-F. (2011). The impact of a theatre performance on mental health service delivery in the context of user involvement. *Dramatherapy, 33*(2), 87–100.

Johnson, D. R. (1982). Developmental approaches to dramatherapy. *Arts in Psychotherapy, 9*, 183–189.

Luft, J., & Ingham, H. (1955). *The Johari window, a graphic model of interpersonal awareness*. Proceedings of the western training laboratory in group development. Los Angeles: UCLA.

Pendzik, S. (1988). Dramatherapy on abuse: A descent to the underworld. *Dramatherapy, 11*(2), 81–92.

Rose, A. M. (Ed.) (1962). *Human behavior and social processes: An interactionist approach*. New York: Houghton Mifflin.

Sajnani, N. (2012). The implicated witness: Towards a relational aesthetic in dramatherapy. *Dramatherapy, 34*(1), 6–21.

Sarbin, T. R. (Ed.) (1986). *Narrative psychology: The storied nature of human conduct*. New York: Praeger.

Stern, D. (2004). *The present moment in psychotherapy and everyday life*. London: W.W. Norton.

Stevens, A. (1990). *On Jung*. London: Routledge.

Van Erven, E. (1988). *Radical people's theatre*. London: Wiley.

Yotis, L. (2002). *Dramatherapy performance and schizophrenia*. Unpublished PhD thesis, University of Hertfordshire.

CHAPTER 14

Personal Theatre and Pedagogy: A Dialectical Process

Anna Seymour

This chapter sets out from a dialectical perspective to address the question: What do we mean by *performing the self* and what pedagogical role might it play as the culmination of training to become a dramatherapist? Since Goffman's (1971) *The Presentation of Self in Everyday Life*, the notion of performance has expanded in many contexts and emerged as a key critical perspective within theatre studies.

Within the field of dramatherapy, performance is used to fulfil a number of purposes. As Renée Emunah (2015) points out in her article in *Drama Therapy Review*, these performances, which include *self-revelatory performance, autobiographical theatre* and perhaps the broadest category *therapeutic theatre,* offer opportunities for healing, personal inquiry, celebration or reflection. The balance or emphasis placed on these processes will be determined by the particular form, those involved, and the discrete boundaries they have set. My purpose here is to make a contribution to the conversation—from what begins as an acknowledgment that within performance there is a persistent/ubiquitous meta-narrative of contradiction. I also argue that contradiction plays a central role in the pedagogical relationship. Just as the therapist works to put herself out of a job or

A. Seymour, PhD, PFHEA, HCPC (✉)
University of Roehampton, London, UK
e-mail: anna.seymour@tiscali.co.uk

the parent secures an attachment in order to allow for healthy separation, the pedagogical relationship embodies a continual exchange within the teacher/student role.

Dialectical praxis embraces the inextricable, reflexive relationship between ideation and its material, embodied manifestation, conception and crafting. The chapter discusses this relationship with reference to the reflections by students on their final performances in the MA Dramatherapy programme at the University of Roehampton in London.

> Students devise and develop a 10-minute solo personal theatre performance which encapsulates and conveys their experience of the training through theatrical metaphor, involving a range of theatrical and dramaturgical techniques and skills. (extract from MA Dramatherapy University of Roehampton Student Handbook)

The author of this chapter conducted informal qualitative research with a group of self-selecting recent graduates, asking them to reflect on their solo performances. The purpose was not to provide any systematic analysis of the process or to produce measurable research outcomes, but to learn more about the students' experience of performing the self. By facilitating these opportunities for self-reflection at some distance from the performances, the author was able to record aspects of the graduates' responses to their own process, in recalling something of what the live experience was like and how it felt to revisit the work, by re-creating a vignette drawn from their original performances. Signed written consent to write about the process was obtained and all quotations taken directly from the graduates are presented in italics.

THE DIALECTICAL PROCESS

The *dialectic* rests on the tension between opposites in relationship, which owe their very existence to the other in both material and abstract senses (for example, a working class cannot exist without a ruling class nor a master without a slave, or vice versa). Yet this is not a system of crude binarisms but the description of a relationship which can be subtly nuanced, and in a state of continual flux and change. These simply stated but deeply complex societal meta-narratives impose themselves within the intimacy of self-reflection and are implicated later when we come to themes of *not good enough* in the performance of the *internal critic*.

The starting point for my analysis can be expressed by a historical figure conceived as a dramatic fictional character:

> My object is not to establish that I was right but to find out if I am... what we discover today we shall wipe off the slate tomorrow and only write it up again once we have again discovered it. And whatever we wish to find we shall regard once found, with particular mistrust... Only when we have failed, have been utterly and hopelessly beaten and are licking our wounds in the profoundest depression, shall we start asking if we weren't right after all. (Bertolt Brecht, 1980, *Galileo,* scene 9, pp. 80–1)

This extract from Bertolt Brecht's *Galileo* describes the dialectic as not only a method of working but also an attitude towards it. Like Brecht's concept of *gestus* (the action, which also embodies an attitude towards the action), the dialectic embraces knowledge, scrutiny, and doubt. Brecht not only uses this conception of gestus in the embodied physical expression of actors, but also extends the idea into the spatial distribution of material objects, emblematic setting and the relationship between actors on stage. Thus, each aspect of the mise-en-scène stands in relationship to its own internal/external makeup (it has a relationship to itself), and at the same time, in relationship to the larger sociopolitical context that informs the construction of the scene in the first place. Embedded in this process is the idea of constructed representation as well as the potential to be in critical relationship with it. Brecht is extracting from the experiences of everyday life and reconceptualising them for the stage. Boundaries on every level are both set and examined.

In the play, Galileo's scientific research challenges the boundaries of existing knowledge, but what counts as knowledge is itself under question, since what is known is also what is allowed to be known under the aegis of the Catholic Church. Galileo stands between material experience and belief systems that are ideologically reinforced. It is of particular significance that the pursuit of this new knowledge involves pain and suffering, a personal process of self-doubt and mistrust. In this drama, the protagonist performer, Galileo, begins from a position of subjective and social knowingness which he challenges over and over and rediscovers. It is through the very pain of going through this process, that knowledge is claimed.

Yet at the same time precisely because this is a ceaseless inquiry there is no settling back into the snug armchair of certainty. Rather there is the messy business, which is familiar to dramatherapists, of 'hopelessly beaten', 'licking wounds' and 'profoundest depression'. There is a constant holding of the dynamic tension between knowledge and ignorance along with a groundedness in the materiality of embodied social experience.

It is precisely these aspects that are engaged in both the process of constructing the performances and in reflecting upon them. In this chapter, I examine how the experiences described by the students and my own observations can be understood through dialectics. It is not an easy process; in the words of Frederic Jameson, 'the dialectic requires you to say everything simultaneously whether you think you can or not' (Jameson, 2007 p. ix). This bold premise points to what the liveness and multilayered simultaneity of performance attempts to capture.

In his unpublished conference presentation on the dialectic, David Barnett (2015) points out that the process has been challenged as deterministic and perpetuating simplistic binaries. However, he supports my argument that such criticisms fail to recognise the philosophical ethos of the dialectic as a dynamic account of flux. It also misses the point that the dialectic is concerned with 'a third thing' (see Rancière below); the relationship itself, which is not just one of contrast or conflict but is, to a greater or lesser extent, in a state of constant mutability, dependent on the balance of power. It is the relationship that is the defining feature of the dialectic, continually being renegotiated in a robust, dynamic and inclusive process.

We could regard dialectics from a methodological perspective as a value-free system drawn from philosophical roots whereby the classical paradigm of thesis/antithesis/synthesis is played out continually. However as soon as this process is contextualised, the specificity of subjective and meta-narratives, as illustrated with reference to *Galileo*, introduce ideological dimensions.

There are further theoretical issues that emerge around the nature of the construction of the self and notions of identity. As Judith Butler, interviewed in 2012, noted:

> When the self, very much alone, tries to reflect on itself...it makes use of a set of conventions, terms, and norms that the self has not authored. These are social conventions that come to us from language and from a broader field

of social signification in which we are all formed. When we start to reflect on ourselves, we do not shed that social formation. It is there in the interstices of our thoughts and even in our idea of what a 'self' should be. So though one can be quite isolated in one's thinking and even physically alone...the social world still mediates our most intimate relations to ourselves. (Pages & Trachman, 2012)

Viewing the political and theoretical developments of the last half-century, from the civil rights movements, to identity struggles embracing gender, sexuality, race, and disability, the sweep of history reveals a movement away from the generalization of collectivity to the fragmentation of specificity. In other words, away from assumptions of shared meaning towards struggles to define and establish uniqueness and difference. This political movement is linked to the theoretical development of post-structuralist thought. At the same time, the need for mechanisms to generate shared meaning and collective agreement has persisted. It is significant that in the field of theatre and performance studies, there has been a turn towards the dialectic as a source of critical renewal, as evidenced by two conferences in the United Kingdom to which I contributed: 'Whither Political Theatre' (University of Cambridge 2014) and 'Performing Dialectics' (Queen Mary University 2015). In the latter context there was expressed a desire to: 'explore whether dialectics can offer performance studies a method of reading the present cultural, theoretical and social moment, in a way that allows for movement, critique and transformation' (Department of Drama, Queen Mary University, London).

Transformation is a word often used in therapeutic practice but in dramatherapy, since our practice is predicated on action, we are aware that the magic of transformation emerges from the careful crafting of the process. In the material that follows, which offers examples of graduates' responses to their solo performances, over and over again the experience of *contradiction* emerges.

Personal Theatre Performances in Training

The performances of self mark the transition from trainee to dramatherapist. The preparation for these solo performances is marked by considerable anxiety as well as anticipation. Excitement is mixed with dread.

Look at me, no don't look at me. I want you to see me, no please don't look.

Immediately contradiction is present in the dynamics of performance—a literal or metaphorical step back or forwards into a space in which the focus of attention is directed towards the performer, an attention that can provoke anxiety for the individual. When the space is delineated by stage lighting it means: '*I can be seen and I am also exposed.*' Yet there is also the potential to respond as if in the game from young childhood—I can't see you so you are not there or as one graduate stated, '*the performance space seems to be blind.*' This tension is played out repeatedly:

- *I am blushing—exposed and nervous and I have a desire to be seen and recognised.*

Themes of exposure are frequently associated with shame and yet the very act of exposure can also be releasing, cathartic and empowering. One graduate described moving through this process as '*affirming.*'

- *Hiding/protecting myself by performing a movement that did not lead to me feeling vulnerable. Detaching slightly. Adopting a persona.*
- *I can pretend that I'm not being watched and this makes me feel safe enough to reveal more.*
- *Stepped in and closed my eyes (warmth) movement—vulnerable? Being seen.*

The themes of both 'being/not being seen' were present:

Perversely, suddenly not wanting to be seen—ambivalence and then wanting to connect, be acknowledged by the others, wanting to check it's OK.

The question of power also emerged:

- *Pull them in. Force power. To be seen requires strength and presence.*
- *Thinking about not being seen... the impulse towards external destruction.*
- *I had a voice in my head saying, 'Can't you tell I don't want to be seen. Go away. GO AWAY!' Fear shame, helplessness.*

Most of the original performances contained a central performative motif that enabled an onstage relationship between performer and object, symbol, or setting, which worked in a classic dramatherapy sense to concretise and externalise the internal process, through use of the projective object. Even if the story was painful, which it invariably was, these dramatic motifs, along with all of the other theatrical conventions employed, enabled the performance of self to take place.

The strength of the metaphors reproduced in their chosen vignettes and the containing boundaries of the performance context supported the performers to fully inhabit and exist within what they did on stage, as the graduates explained in their reflections:

- *The memory of when I am a three-and-a-half-year-old where my mother put her head on my lap and I felt myself become her mother; the duality of being both praised and berated at the same time when I was six... understanding the dramaturgy of my performance gave me the opportunity to build the puppet of my mother... I think the confrontation with the performing element which awoke 'the actress' inside of me was therapeutic.*
- *My breath was my friend.*
- *Creating a suitable metaphor was a hard task... it soon became clear that I needed to perform my piece as myself.*
- *I wanted to root the performance in the body of me and what this mapped and represented. A large red birthmark on my left leg has long been a defining feature of my body and how I feel about myself. The more I thought about it, and reflected on it the more I realised how my birthmark was a metaphor for all the things I wanted to expose and celebrate about myself and my journey on the course. It represents a history of rejection and bullying, of fear and shame, the things I hide because I am scared of what others might think and also my uniqueness, beauty and flaw.*
- *I made a conscious decision not to use music or theatrical aids as I wanted the performance to be about my body, vulnerable, in the empty space and what this held for me and the audience.*

The themes that emerged indicated the stories that each performer wanted to tell the audience. They made choices about what they wanted to be seen. At the same time, however much control performers exercise over what they chose to show, they cannot fully control what can be seen and this was expressed directly in the process group:

- *I feel like I've been more seen than I see myself.*

I would argue there is an implicit dialectical pedagogy embedded in the performance relationship but, as with all dialectical process, the outcomes may not always be known.

The Pedagogical Process of Personal Theatre Performance

The Brechtian... delight in learning, lie(s) ultimately in the gestus of showing. The opening scene of Galileo is, after all, less a mimesis of scientific knowledge... than it is a representation of how you go about transmitting and conveying such knowledge... teaching is thus showing... the dramatic representation of teaching is the showing of showing, the showing of how you show and demonstrate. (Jameson, 2000, p. 91)

One of my contentions in this chapter is that the performance of self in the academic context is multilayered in its pedagogy. It focuses the individual student's attention towards crafting aspects of his or her experience through theatrical aesthetics that cannot take place without reference to the theoretical aspects of the training. This creates a level of detachment that allows for reflection on choices of form and content to be presented. By virtue of this dimension, there is a further layer of pedagogy where the performer teaches the audience about what—and how—they want the audience to know.

In the following example, the graduate adopted a precise approach to staging where the delineation of upstage and downstage areas allowed for different embodied presentations of self:

- *The idea for my performance was my relationship with my inner critic... to find a way to not only present to others how I feel my internal narrative impacts my emotions and experiences, but also to find a way to externalise that experience for myself. I wanted to keep the performance very simple... making the introduction of my inner critic (to both audience and in many ways, to myself) very simple and clear edged.*

The careful construction of the performance contained painful material that was, as she put it, 'poisonous and destructive' as evidenced here:

- *You're failing. You're failing to impress, you're failing to take risks, you're failing to be interesting. You've failed.*
- *It's done. [pause... raises finger]*
- *You see, now, she's blocking. [takes deep breath]*
- *She's taken that deep breath, she's wrapping around that skin, that façade that says she's coping, she's happy, she's light, she's airy—she's rotting. She's dead, dumb rotting meat.*

Yet this inner critic figure enabled what the graduate described as a cathartic experience to take place:

- *It felt exciting and stimulating, adrenaline inducing. I utterly loved it. I felt powerful and interesting and LOUD, loud enough to be heard! (perhaps this is something to do with the character of my inner critic—normally it is only heard by me—perhaps it relished being able to be heard by others... to be able to express what this critic character inside me has to say felt like a release... to air (these thoughts) meant I could put the weight down—even if just for a few moments.*

Members of the process group expressed contradictory reactions to each other's performances:

- *There's a conflict in me feeling how brilliant you are in your self-despising.*
- *I had a physical response that can't be translated into words.*

At the same time, comments on containment, self-preservation, protection, and acceptance point to an appreciation by witnesses that the performer is making distinct choices and guiding the experience.

The personal value of the experience to the graduate is perhaps best expressed thus:

- *I had a real physical sense of my own courage.*

As Roger Grainger (2013) states: 'The discomfort of theatre occurs in varying degrees of intensity throughout a range of dramatic conventions; it would be hard to see how there could be any emotional satisfaction without it' (p. 82).

The dialectic both identifies and engages the contradictory tensions of relationship. If the dialectical relationship (for instance, I can know myself through knowing you) is denied, if the individual is trapped in the idea of the immutability of self, or an unassailable sense of personal uniqueness, we reach the aloneness of fragmentation, patronisation, narcissism, isolation, and stuckness. Yet the purpose of drama is to create *shared* meaning and indeed the whole basis of performance rests on the idea that there is an audience, which, for all its plurality, can embrace a performative vocabulary. The dialectic resonates with the core theatrical principles of *engagement* and, to conclude, I turn to the role of audience for the performance of self.

REFLECTIONS ON THE ROLE OF AUDIENCE AS WITNESS

Theatre director Di Trevis describes the unique nature of every audience and recommends to actors and directors to 'allow the audience to teach you... about the play' (2012, p. 128). This recommendation captures the aliveness of the performance itself and recommends receptivity to the nuances of audience reaction. The exchange between stage and audience is both inevitable and necessary.

In the words of two of the graduates:

- *... being witnessed made it terrifying, but it was this that made it powerful.*
- *Being witnessed was a fundamental part in my journey towards healing and growing both as a person and as a dramatherapist.*

In his 2009 book, *The Emancipated Spectator,* the philosopher Jacques Rancière examines the dialectical role of the audience. Rancière's views have become significant in a number of fields (politics, critical theory and aesthetics) and could be of use in dramatherapy. The eminent dramatherapist and actor Roger Grainger describes theatre as 'a worthwhile embarrassment' (2013, p. 81) which is 'characterised by discomfiture, the emotional disturbance suffered by personages in the play itself (and the actors impersonating them of course) and the disquiet which this arouses in the audience' (p. 81). Rancière's (2009) initial discussion is already familiar to theatre scholars. He is concerned with what appear to be the negative power relations between the stage and audience, regarding *viewing* as the opposite of *knowing*, where there is an ignorance of the process of production, and that viewing is the opposite of *acting*, as the viewers are passive in their seats. He sums this up as 'The spectator is separated from the ability to know and the power to act' (p. 3).

To alleviate matters, he then cites Brechtian alienation (encouraging the capacity to judge) and Artaud's (1974) *vital energy in ritual* (encouraging the capacity to viscerally engage) as potentials for the spectator's role. In each case the audience still remains 'in its place' (Rancière, 2009, p. 7). Although he does not refer to more contemporary examples such as Boal's (1979) shifting the role of spectator to *spect-actor*, nor to the many experiments with participation, reconfiguration of space, and site-specific performance that have gone on since the late 1960s, Rancière poses some delicate arguments about how the role of spectator can be reconceived. And in doing so engages in a number of ideas that are central to witnessing in the dramatherapy process, as well as relating to the current discussion of the dialectical process.

Rancière is concerned with the individual subject in the apparent community of the audience, claiming, 'Theatre remains the only place where the audience confronts itself as a collective' (2009, p. 5); yet this is where an implicit dialectic is engaged. He sees the emancipated role of the spectator as one in which 'the spectator also acts, like the pupil or scholar. She observes, selects, compares, interprets. She links what she sees to a host of other things that she has seen on other stages, in other kinds of place. She composes her own poem with the elements of the poem before her' (2009, p. 13).

In a 2011 interview, published in the collection of essays, *Reading Rancière* (Bowman & Stamp, 2011, p. 244), Rancière states, 'There is always a plurality of ways of constituting a community, just as there is in defining the singularity of an individual.' He also refers to 'the third thing that is owned by no one' (Rancière, 2009, p. 15). This is the new relationship that exists as the product of a dialectical tension—between the knowledge, experiences and vocabularies of the performer and audience, between the knowing and unknowing.

In the liminality of this unknown space there is considerable risk, as described by a graduate:

- *I wanted to be, however that manifested itself in the moment, with the awareness that this would also be a being with, an unmasked meeting between the audience and myself. I feel I did achieve this, terrified as I was of it, and tempted as I was to shy away from this challenge... scared as I was I felt capable by the end of the course of taking that moment. What I did not expect was to enjoy it. My fear was gone. The audience felt warm and I felt warm towards them... happy just to be there... a tangible experience which I can take away and treasure.*

The performance cannot take place without an audience. As Rancière discusses, theatre makers have worked to reposition the role of audience in relation to the stage actor—from Grotowski's (1975) eviscerated sacrificial actor (Kumiega, 1985) who evokes the rituals of Catholicism, to Boal's (1979) politically charged reconfiguration of the relationship.

In the context of the performances of self described in this chapter, the actors prepared to meet the audience, however it presented itself. There was no conscious process of using theatrical skills to *act* but rather using theatrical skills to be in performance. There could be certain assumptions about empathy and kindness, given that the audience was made up of families and various supporters. Nonetheless the prevailing attitude amongst the graduates was one of wanting to stay with showing themselves through performance and adopting faith in the process that, by doing so with authenticity, personal goals would be achieved.

CONCLUSION

- *I remember the moment just before the final blackout; I felt genuinely triumphant, elated, energised and buoyed up by what I had done.*

In training to be a dramatherapist, we acknowledge that we would not expect others to tread a path that we ourselves feared to tread. We invite our clients to step into the unknown, bringing with them all they know about the pain of their lived experience. In the solo performances of self described in this chapter, the trainee dramatherapists bring into a public space their cumulative insights into their own process, discovering and re-committing to an engagement with the healing, contradictory forces of making theatre.

REFERENCES

Artaud, A. (1974) [1932]. The theatre of cruelty (First manifesto), In *Collected works*, vol. 4, trans. Victor Corti. London: Calder.

Barnett, D. (2015). *Brecht in practice: Theatre, theory and performance*. London: Bloomsbury.

Boal, A. (1979). *The theatre of the oppressed*. Trans. Charles A. & Maria-Odilia Leal McBride. London: Pluto Press.

Brecht, B. (1980). *Life of Galileo*. London: Methuen.

Bowman, P., & Stamp, R. (Eds.) (2011). *Reading Rancière*. London: Continuum.

Emunah, R. (2015). Self-revelatory performance: A form of drama therapy and theatre. *Drama Therapy Review, 1*(1), 71–85.

Goffman, E. (1971). *The presentation of self in everyday life*. London: Penguin.

Grainger, R. (2013). *Nine ways the theatre affects our lives*. Lampeter: Edward Mellen Press.

Grotowski, J. (1975). *Towards a poor theatre*. London: Eyre Methuen.

Kumiega, J. (1985). *The theatre of Grotowski*. London: Methuen.

Jameson, F. (2000). *Brecht and method*. London: Verso.

Jameson, F. (2007). *The modernist papers*. London: Verso.

Pages, C., & Trachman, M. (2012). Analytics of power: An interview with Judith Butler. http://www.booksandideas.net

Ranciére, J. (2009). *The emancipated spectator*. London: Verso.

Trevis, D. (2012). *Becoming a director: A life in theatre*. London: Routledge/ Taylor and Francis.

CHAPTER 15

Autobiographical Therapeutic Theatre with Older People with Dementia

Dovrat Harel

During the last two decades we have witnessed extensive change in the perception of dementia care. This change has been rooted in the ideas of Kitwood (2007), which were later conceptualized as the 'person-centered dementia care approach' (Woods, 1999). Kitwood advocated to stop focusing on the illness and on the tendency to depersonalize and disempower people with dementia, adopting instead a positive attitude that takes into account each person's individuality and uniqueness, including his or her life story and current coping resources (Bryden, 2002). Kitwood laid the foundation for a revolution in dementia care, creating a shift from the medical model to the psychosocial model of practice (Knocker, 2001). The 'person-centered dementia care approach' seeks to illuminate the person's capabilities and preserved abilities instead of their difficulties and losses; it encourages the expression of individuality in a social context as opposed to the common tendency to withdraw (Bryden, 2002). This conceptual change reinforced the use of creative methods for helping people with dementia and their caregivers. Research about the correlation between aging and creativity (Baird, 1996; Cohen, 2001, 2006) and the

D. Harel (✉)
Bar-Ilan University, Ramat Gan, Israel

Haifa University, Haifa, Israel
e-mail: dovrat_harel@yahoo.com

© The Author(s) 2016
S. Pendzik et al. (eds.), *The Self in Performance*,
DOI 10.1057/978-1-137-53593-1_15

particular contribution of creativity to older people with dementia (Gross et al., 2015; Killick, 2013; Marshall, 2013; Schweitzer & Bruce, 2008), support the use of creative arts therapies as an effective, fulfilling, and valuable tool with this population.

Previous drama therapy and theatre group work with older people with dementia has shown the particular contribution of spontaneous play to life enrichment and to the adjustment to changes (Gay & Perlstein, 2008; Johnson, 1986; Knocker, 2001; Langley, 1987). The potential for integrating reminiscence therapy and theatre has been examined by several drama therapy and theatre projects. Some of these involved professional actors who transformed the seniors' memories into theatrical pieces that were then presented to them as well as to other seniors (Langley, 1987; Schweitzer, 2007). Other programs emphasized the importance of role playing, introducing the participation of volunteers, youth, students or caregivers in the drama groups for older people, thus stressing the intergenerational principle (Gay & Perlstein, 2008).

As a drama therapist working for many years with older people with dementia, I developed a therapeutic model to help them achieve a sense of well-being and 'ego integrity' (Erikson, 1968). The model adheres to the life course approach, which suggests that people continue to develop and grow throughout the whole of their lives (Holstein & Gubrium, 2000). It combines theory and practice, integrating some of the new insights in the field of dementia care and creativity, such as narrative gerontology, life review and reminiscence, with drama therapy.

Most dementia illnesses are progressive; early symptoms differ markedly from those in later stages (Draper, 2004). The use of Autobiographical Therapeutic Theatre is relevant for older adults with early stage dementia (also termed mild dementia). These people suffer from short-term memory impairment and some personality changes. They may function independently for the most part, but require assistance with specific activities. Although needing encouragement in order to be socially active, they usually experience great enjoyment when offered reassurance in a safe environment. Therefore, group work is an ideal setting in which they can establish meaningful interpersonal relationships, develop a sense of belonging (Schweitzer & Bruce, 2008), and experience the empowering effect of mutuality, when given the opportunity to care for and support others, instead of being cast in the passive role of the recipients (Haight & Gibson, 2005).

I use *autobiographical therapeutic theatre* (ATT) in the framework of drama therapy, progressing from process-oriented to performance-oriented (Bailey, 2009) or performance-based modalities (Snow, 2009). Rather than being limited to verbal expression, participants explore their past experiences through improvisation, making use of a wide variety of self-expressive methods. The fact that life memories are taken to the domain of dramatic reality enables participants to actually awaken and bring them to life (not only to share them verbally), while at the same time effecting a movement from 'teller' to 'actor'. This role shift involves the use of many senses simultaneously, thus making it particularly valuable for people with dementia (Schweitzer, 2007).

As group members act together, portraying themselves in their own stories and playing secondary roles in others people's experiences, a strong supportive net of stories and characters is weaved, increasing group cohesion. In my experience, the dramatization of life stories contributes in turn to honing memory: When the senses are stimulated and the past is revived in the here and now, details become clearer, life experiences acquire multidimensional status, and various interpretations become available. This process enables participants to expand their perspective on the course of their life, revisiting the different roles they played, the positions they held, and the relationships they had. They recall their strengths and coping mechanisms from the past, and these are reassimilated into their current identity. As the process moves towards the performance-oriented stages, involving rehearsal and production, they begin to deconstruct their current image as people with dementia, and to reconstruct new and more powerful identities (Snow et al., 2003).

The process is informed by *Narrative Gerontology* (an approach that implements the narrative paradigm in the field of gerontology), which is based on the ontology of the human being as storyteller and even *Homo-Narrans* (Myerhoff, 1978), and on the life-as-story metaphor. Narrative gerontology perceives the need to tell life stories during old age as natural and universal, and assumes that older people with dementia are biographically active and have narrative agency (Kenyon et al., 2011). This approach believes that older people can construct and reconstruct their self-identity through the action of telling their life stories (McAdams, 1996).

Furthermore, my work implements *Life-Review* and *Reminiscence* techniques, which are informed by Robert Butler's (1963) ideas. In his view, as people approach the end of their lives, they seek to put their experiences in perspective, resolve past conflicts, grieve losses and changes, forgive themselves and others, celebrate successes, and feel a sense of closure. In contrast to the tendency espoused by many health care professionals (and society in general), who regarded reminiscence as a symptom of senility or other types of mental illness (Kuntz, 2007), Butler (1963) recommended encouraging older adults to take part in structured reminiscence and life-reviewing activities, in order to support this natural need and promote its aims. The advantage of reminiscence work with older people with dementia is that it provides them with the opportunity to use their long-term memory, which is still intact in the early stages of dementia, rather than their short-term memory, which is the first mechanism to be damaged. The memories, therefore, are a kind of treasure. They have the power to connect people to the best moments in their life, and at the same time provide a sense of ability and accomplishment.

Project Description

I have used ATT with several groups in a day care center for senior citizens in Israel. Each group included between four and six older adults with early stage dementia and an equivalent number of young drama therapy students from the Graduate School of Creative Arts Therapies at Haifa University. The groups were composed of pairs: each student worked individually with a specific senior citizen. Many activities also involved the group as a whole. This setting gave all the individuals maximum attention, while emphasizing aspects of belonging to a group and concurrently encouraging the utilization of social skills. The groups met once a week for 90 minutes, for a period of seven months. A digital camera was used to document special moments during the process. This documentation, together with other creative products, was used later as 'memory supporters', to reflect on the personal process. The process of our work progresses through five stages within the series of sessions:

Stage One: Reminiscence and Life Stories Elaboration

This stage aims to conjure up a wide range of life stories and a comprehensive and meaningful self-presentation. After two introductory sessions, the group focuses on reminiscence and life review processes followed by drama therapy exercises. Each session deals with a specific theme, including childhood, adolescence, marriage, and becoming parents, or issues such as life-achievements, career, hobbies, and leisure. The sessions in this stage are generally constructed according to the following sub-stages:

Warm-up and Memory Stimulation

The sessions usually begin with singing. Since this skill remains intact well into the first stage of dementia, it provides a sense of ability and enjoyment (Aldridge, 2000). In addition, songs from the participants' past elicit memories and encourage spontaneous responses in the group (Dassa & Amir, 2014). The songs are connected to the reminiscence subjects. Subsequently, we use another activity that introduces the session's subject while simultaneously stimulating memory. For example, when dealing with childhood memories, we may begin with some childhood games. This warm-up stimulates long-term memory and spontaneously elicits life stories.

Life Stories Gathering

At this point members are asked to sit in pairs—students and seniors. The students encourage the seniors to tell them their life stories around the main issue. All stories are acceptable: there is no right or wrong in our work. Sometimes, when it's difficult for the seniors to recall a memory from a specific theme, the students are asked to share their own memories as triggers for the memories of their senior counterpart.

Life Stories Elaboration and Dramatization

Through skilled and sensitive listening, emphasis is placed on particular details that have the potential to provide the narrators with a positive attitude towards themselves. Sometimes this perspective is explicitly communicated by the narrator, while in other cases it has to be read between the lines. When necessary, the students ask clarifying questions in order to retrieve more details. Next, each pair prepares a short dramatic presentation of the story that expresses its positive aspects. Whenever the presentation involves more than two participants, other group members are invited to play in the scene, thus the group acts together as a unit. If people share stories with conflicting or emotionally disturbing content, distancing techniques such as *Playback Theatre* (Fox, 1994; Salas, 1996) or *Dramatic Resonances* (Pendzik, 2008) are used in order to gain aesthetic distance from the story and encourage the person to look at it from a new and wider perspective.

In this context I would like to explain the concept of the *enlarging positive mirror*. This notion refers to the use of drama therapy interventions that can reveal and reflect back the positive aspects present in a story, even if they are only implicitly communicated. Inspired by the positive psychology, we seek to increase an awareness of achievements, accomplishments, capabilities, good decisions, successes, and any other factors contributing to the construction of a positive self-image. Some people tell life stories with a clear, positive emphasis while others tend to conceal positive aspects. Sometimes the positive content is inaccessible to the person, as a result of sad and harmful experiences—a characteristic of many traumatic life stories. The enlarging positive mirror provides a constructive option in these cases, as, fortunately, many difficult experiences, even the traumatic ones, contain positive aspects as well—albeit appearing as minor details or hardly expressed in the dominant narrative. With highly sensitive active listening, it is possible to become aware of descriptions that indicate significant strengths—for example, a wise decision made at a critical moment. Using 'the enlarging positive mirror' doesn't mean changing the story: the drama therapist tries to remain true to the original story, while concurrently reflecting the positive, reassuring, and consoling aspects of it within the framework of dramatic reality. The plot remains faithful to the original narrative, but some of its silent voices are spoken out loud, and details that might have been perceived as insignificant become more central and meaningful.

Processing and Closure

All group members, young and old, share their experience from the session. The seniors are asked how they feel about their stories and their dramatization, and specific attention is given to their self-perception following the process.

Stage Two: Story Selection

When many significant stories have been told, the group moves on to the next stage. This turning point is marked by one session that is devoted to choosing the stories that are going to be included in the performance. The session involves a review of the entire first stage and a recapitulation of the stories that had been told, accompanied by pictures and other creative products that were produced throughout the meetings, in order to help the participants remember the context and support their memory. Sitting in pairs to recap, the students help the seniors to choose one or two that they would like to share with the audience. Students must be aware of ethical considerations, for if the seniors have some difficulty with their judgment skills, they may have to help them choose stories that present them in a positive and respectable manner. Stories that contain a highly sensitive or intimate content, for example, should be reconsidered.

The drama therapist and the students then write a script of an original play, trying to stay as faithful as possible to the participants' choices and preferences, and consulting them regarding the script and any changes they wish to make. This approach is not to be underestimated, since people with dementia often experience being controlled by their caregivers without being granted many opportunities for choice and mastery. In order to emphasize this therapeutic intervention while taking members' cognitive limitations into consideration, every personal story in the play is created so that it stands on its own, while the script also links all the stories in a cohesive sequence that connects them aesthetically. For example, in the play *Memories with a Cup of Coffee*, there was a framing story of four friends who meet every afternoon for coffee, and during their conversation, the memories come up and are performed.

As exemplified by this play, the model maintains two parallel axes: the collective and the individual. The collective axis represents the group process, aimed at providing participants with a sense of belonging and of keeping them socially active. In addition, it gives elderly people with dementia (a stigmatized group) an opportunity to have voice to express themselves (Emunah & Johnson, 1983) and to bring the audience into greater proximity to them (Sajnani, 2012). The individual axis focuses on the personal content of the life stories and on self-presentation, leading to positive self-identity construction.

Stage Three: Rehearsals

From this point on, the group begins to work as a theatre group and to rehearse the play. However, as I have already mentioned, the therapeutic goals are paramount: A supportive atmosphere is promoted and pressure is always avoided. In order to prevent participant burnout and fatigue, the rehearsal stage does not exceed five meetings.

This stage is generally characterized by reinforcing the involvement of the participants—older and younger. As the rehearsals progress, people miss fewer meetings than was the case in previous stages; they often express mutual concern and seem to bond as a group. I have noticed that during the rehearsals period, older members tend to look much more vital, and some even adopt a proactive attitude, such as voluntarily bringing objects and pictures from home. The feedback I receive from the staff at this stage often includes positive changes in the participant's behavior and mood. I also have received similar feedback directly from participants. For example, a woman, who was generally moody and used to complain of fatigue, stated that since she had begun rehearsing the play, she was sleeping much better and feeling much more alert. She also added that the headaches she had suffered from had stopped, attributing these positive changes to taking part in our project.

While rehearsing the play, life stories are further elaborated and more details from long-term memory emerge. Sometimes these are followed by reactions of surprise, as these memories were dormant, and are retrieved only as the stories are repeatedly dramatized. During the rehearsals, participants occasionally request changes to the text, emphasizing some aspects, leaving out specific parts, or adding information. Since one of the main goals is to encourage a sense of mastery, these requests are consistently met. In this way, the performed stories gradually attain their final form in a dialogical process.

The rehearsal stage symbolizes the willingness to share personal stories with people outside the group. This process is reinforced when we begin to work in the space where the performance will take place. In order to establish a safe space and reduce anxiety, we use some memory supporters—particularly music. Music aids participants to follow the sequence of the play. We found it very valuable to integrate a musician (usually a pianist) in the rehearsal stage (and, of course, in the performance). We often choose a specific song for each participant, using it as a resonance of the dramatized life story (Pendzik, 2008). Generally, participants know a song that the story reminds them of, but if they don't, some options are offered. The musician adapts the rhythm to the participants' physical abilities, which helps to reduce pressure and anxiety of not keeping up, and gives them a sense of accomplishment. We also use some visual 'memory supporters', such as a large poster at the back of the stage with a list of the stories, objects and stage props that remind the participants what should be performed.

Stage Four: The Performance

The process results in an autobiographical therapeutic performance that is enacted in front of relatives, friends, staff, and professionals in the community. The group members experience the power of performing on stage, while feeling 'embraced' by an empathic and supportive audience (Sajnani, 2012; Snow et al., 2003). Goffman's (1959) notion that people transmit personal and social identity in interpersonal interaction is tangibly present in the experience of performing in front of an audience. As Emunah and Johnson (1983) stated, the direct encounter with the audience is an opportunity for the participants to confirm the development of the self-image that they attained during the rehearsals.

The senior members, who often experience a low self-image as they see themselves as old and cognitively impaired, realize that many people have come to watch them and to acknowledge their past, getting a reinforcing message of being significant and valued. This act of expression and affirmation promotes growth and positive change (Mackay, 1996). Speaking about the thin line between artist and person in self-revelatory and in therapeutic theatre performances, Emunah (1994) claims that performers 'are applauded not only for their creative achievement, but for the process they have been through in creating it, for their courage to reveal themselves, and for who they are as people' (p. 289). She adds that the participants experience not only accomplishment but also acceptance, which is intensified when the performers are socially stigmatized people and their identity has been presented to the audience.

The audience takes also an important part during the performance. For instance, they may be asked to sing along with the live music accompaniment. These are the songs that participants have previously selected, which were integrated as *dramatic resonances* (Pendzik, 2008) and as memory supporters (to indicate when they need to prepare for the next story). While the actors get organized on the backstage, they clearly hear the audience singing their songs. This action emphasizes the reciprocity, as performers benefit from the audience's empathy, while simultaneously they bestow 'upon the audience the gift of inspired live theatrical art' (Emunah, 2015, p. 80).

All the group members, both students and seniors, participate actively in the performance. The older people portray themselves as children, teenagers or young adults, while other members of the group play secondary roles. The students make sure that the seniors' comfort and well-being are maintained during the show, and special attention is paid to reducing pressure and sustaining a relaxed atmosphere. As a performative modality, the quality of the product is important, yet the pursuit of good artistic theatre is not at the expense of the participant's therapeutic needs (Landy & Montgomery, 2012; Mitchell, 1994).

Stage Five: Closure and Follow-Up

After the performance the group meets for several weeks in order to reflect on the communal journey, process the experience and find ways of integrating it in their daily lives. Participants share their experiences from the performance, reflecting also on the meaning of the entire project and on what they will take with them in the future. This part of the process links the past (the memories and life stories), the present (the awareness of current experiences) and the future (what they will take from the process)—establishing a sense of ego integrity though continuity. This is illustrated, for instance, by one of the participants, who told us that as a result of the project she now understands how much she accomplished in her life, and proudly added: 'Now I can say that I was also an actress!' From the perspective of the model, this implies that she had accomplished a step towards acquiring or integrating a new role.

But alongside the satisfaction and sense of accomplishment, following the performance participants may experience symptoms of post-performance depression (Emunah, 1994) and be overwhelmed with feelings of emptiness and loss. Anticipating the separation from the group may exacerbate the potential for depression and reactivate some negative aspects of old age. Emunah (1994) states that this is another therapeutic stage, in which the greatest challenge is to integrate and assimilate personal and collective accomplishments. In order to help alleviate the emptiness of the ending, each participant is given an album containing pictures from the entire project, including the performance. This album is offered as a closing ritual, and as a kind of *transitional object* (Winnicott, 1971), serving as a memento from the process.

Once the project is completed, I continue in some way to be the bond between the project and the participants' return to daily routine. I come to the center to accompany the seniors in a more informal way, and make sure that they are well adjusted to the routine now that the group meetings are over. During my weekly visits I have personal conversations with them in order to ensure a sense of continuance and holding.

In addition, the staff at the Day Center is instructed to support the process and carry it on, as witnesses, by mentioning the insights, recalling the emotions generated by the project, and offering their feedback whenever they notice that people need reinforcement. I ask them to continue to echo the life stories presented at the performance among the participants in order to help them to integrate this experience in their normal lives. The staff and the families not only fulfill the role of companion witnesses of the performance: They also embody, concretely as well as symbolically, the participants' daily life; and, as such, they have an important task in carrying on the continuity of the new perspectives achieved.

According to Sajnani (2012), responses of greater proximity between the audience and performers reflect *relational aesthetics* in drama therapy. Witnessing the performances is also beneficial to the families. Watching the performance and sharing life stories from such a gratifying perspective enables relatives to view the elderly person in a more positive light. More than once, people have approached me after the performance and expressed how the experience changed the way they viewed their parent or partner; and this impact on relatives resonates over a long period of time. For instance, the daughter of one of the elderly participants whom I met long after the performance, told me that whenever she hears 'her mother's song' on the radio, she cries, remembering how she had coped bravely with her hardships, as depicted in the play.

Conclusion

As implemented, the model utilized drama therapy students; yet with proper supervision and guidance, other professionals or volunteers who have an affinity to applied or social forms of theatre could participate as assistants. I discovered that the intergenerational presence is crucial: The interaction between older people and the younger generation (students) returns the seniors to their cultural position as the 'elders of the congregation'—a role that was well rooted in our culture and is imperative to revive in our day. The elders enjoy giving the younger participants advice from their life experience, express their knowledge and impart their wisdom. In drama therapy terms, the older participants expand their role system (Landy, 2009) and experience a more empowering position than that of confused and marginalized older people. These benefits can be added to the model's previously mentioned advantages, making it a comprehensive and highly effective model for older people with dementia.

References

Aldridge, D. (2000). Overture: It's not what you do but the way you do it. In D. Aldridge (Ed.), *Music therapy in dementia care* (pp. 9–32). London: Jessica Kingsley Publishers.

Bailey, S. (2009). Performance in drama therapy. In D. Johnson & R. Emunah (Eds.), *Current approaches in drama therapy* (pp. 374–389). Springfield, IL: C. C. Thomas.

Baird, C. M. (1996). *Creative aging: A meaning-making perspective.* New York: Norton.

Bryden, C. (2002). A person-centred approach to counselling, psychotherapy and rehabilitation of people diagnosed with dementia in the early stages. *Dementia, 1*(2), 141–156.

Butler, N. R. (1963). The life review: An interpretation of reminiscence in old age. *Psychiatry Journal for the Study of Interpersonal Processes, 26,* 65–76.

Cohen, G. D. (2001). *The creative age: Awakening human potential in the second half of life.* New York: Quill.

Cohen, G. D. (2006). Research on creativity and aging: The positive impact of the arts on health and illness. *Generations, 30*(1), 7–15.

Dassa, A., & Amir, D. (2014). The role of singing familiar songs in encouraging conversation among people with middle to late stage Alzheimer's disease. *Journal of Music Therapy, 51*(2), 131–153.

Draper, B. (2004). *Dealing with dementia: A guide to Alzheimer's disease and other dementias.* Crow's Nest, NSW: Allen & Unwin.

Emunah, R. (1994). *Acting for real: Drama therapy process, technique, and performance.* New York and London: Brunner-Mazel; Routledge.

Emunah, R. (2015). Self-revelatory performance: A form of drama therapy and theatre. *Drama Therapy Review, 1*(1), 71–85.

Emunah, R., & Johnson, D. (1983). The impact of theatrical performance on the self-images of psychiatric patients. *Arts in Psychotherapy, 10,* 233–239.

Erikson, E. H. (1968). *Identity, youth and crisis.* New York: W.W. Norton.

Fox, J. (1994). *Acts of service: spontaneity, commitment, tradition in the nonscripted theatre.* New York: Tusitala Press.

Gay, H., & Perlstein, S. (2008). Creativity matters: Arts and aging in America. *Monograph. Americans for the Arts.* September, Retrieved July 29, 2015, from https://www.giarts.org/sites/default/files/Monograph_Creativity-Matters-Arts-and-Aging-in-America.pdf

Goffman, E. (1959). *The presentation of self in everyday life.* New York: Anchor Books Doubleday.

Gross, S. M., Danilova, D., Vandehey, M. A., & Diekhoff, G. M. (2015). Creativity and dementia: Does artistic activity affect well-being beyond the art class? *Dementia, 14*(1), 27–46.

Haight, B., & Gibson, F. (2005). Introduction. In B. Haight & F. Gibson (Eds.), *Working with older adults: Group process and techniques* (pp. 3–5). Mississauga and London: Jones and Bartlett Publishers.

Holstein, J. A., & Gubrium, J. F. (2000). *Constructing the life course* (2nd ed.). New York: General Hall.

Johnson, D. R. (1986). The developmental method in drama therapy: Group treatment with elderly. *Arts in Psychotherapy, 13*, 17–33.

Kenyon, G., Bohlmeijer, E., & Randall, W. L. (2011). Preface. In G. Kenyon, E. Bohlmeijer, & W. L. Randall (Eds.), *Storying later life: Issues, investigations and interventions in narrative gerontology* (pp. xiii–xviii). New York: Oxford University Press.

Killick, J. (2013). *Playfulness and dementia: A practice guide.* London: Jessica Kingsley Publications.

Kitwood, T. (2007). Tom Kitwood on dementia—A reader and critical commentary. C. Baldwin & A. Capstick (Eds.). New York: Open University Press.

Knocker, S. (2001). A meeting of worlds: Play and metaphor in dementia care and dramatherapy. *Dramatherapy, 23*(2), 4–9.

Kuntz, J. A. (2007). The life story matrix. In J. A. Kuntz & F. G. Soltys (Eds.), *Transformational reminiscence: Life story work* (pp. 1–16). New York: Springer.

Landy, R. (2009). Role theory and the role method of drama therapy. In D. Johnson & R. Emunah (Eds.), *Current approaches in drama therapy* (pp. 65–88). Springfield, IL: C. C. Thomas.

Landy, R., & Montgomery, D. T. (2012). *Theatre for change: Education, social action and therapy.* London and New York: Palgrave Macmillan.

Langley, D. (1987). Dramatherapy with elderly people. In S. Jennings (Ed.), *Dramatherapy: Theory and practice for teachers and clinicians* (pp. 233–256). London: Jessica Kingsley.

MacKay, B. (1996). Brief drama therapy and the collective creation. In A. Gersie (Ed.), *Dramatic approaches to brief therapy* (pp. 161–174). London: Jessica Kingsley Publications.

Marshall, K. (2013). *Puppetry in dementia care: Connecting through creativity and joy.* London: Jessica Kingsley Publishers.

McAdams, D. P. (1996). Narrating the self in adulthood. In E. Birren, G. M. Kenyon, J. E. Ruth, J. J. F. Schroots, & T. Svensson (Eds.), *Aging and biography: Explorations in adult development* (pp. 131–148). New York: Springer.

Mitchell, S. (1994). The theatre of self-expression: A 'therapeutic theatre' model of drama therapy. In S. Jennings, A. Cattanach, S. Mitchell, A. Chesner, & B. Meldrum (Eds.), *The handbook of drama therapy* (pp. 41–57). London: Routledge.

Myerhoff, B. (1978). *Number our days.* New York: Simon & Schuster.

Pendzik, S. (2008). Dramatic resonances: A technique of intervention in drama therapy, supervision, and training. *Arts in Psychotherapy, 35*, 217–223.

Sajnani, N. (2012). The implicated witness: Towards relational aesthetic in drama-therapy. *Dramatherapy, 34*(1), 6–21.

Salas, J. (1996). *Improvising real life: Personal story in playback theatre.* New York: Tusitala Press.

Schweitzer, P. (2007). *Reminiscence theatre: Making theatre from memories.* London: Jessica Kingsley Publishers.

Schweitzer, P., & Bruce, E. (2008). *Remembering yesterday, caring today – Reminiscence in dementia care.* London and Philadelphia: Jessica Kingsley Publishers.

Snow, S. (2009). Ritual/theatre/therapy. In D. Johnson & R. Emunah (Eds.), *Current approaches in drama therapy* (2nd ed., pp. 44–117). Springfield, IL: C.C. Thomas.

Snow, S., D'Amico, M., & Tanguay, D. (2003). Therapeutic theatre and well-being. *Arts in Psychotherapy, 30*(2), 73–82.

Winnicott, D. W. (1971). *Playing and reality.* London: Tavistock.

Woods, B. (1999). The person in dementia care. *Generations, 23*(3), 35–39.

CHAPTER 16

The Unheard Stories of Those Forgotten Behind Bars in Lebanon

Zeina Daccache

Working as a drama therapist in various settings in Lebanon, I have directed plays with marginalized groups based on their personal experiences, and witnessed the healing power of Self-Revelatory Performance not only for the targeted groups but also for the Lebanese audience: that is, for society as a whole. The work has had the intention—and the effect—of challenging the unjust laws applied in Lebanon against prison inmates, migrant domestic workers, and other beneficiaries, who for the first time here, reflecting on their own lives, stand up before numerous audiences (including governmental figures), and bare their personal stories to heal their own wounds—and those of their community. This chapter tells a tale of self-advocacy, as these marginalized groups hold up a mirror to Lebanese society, implicating it in the oppression that often leads to crime, chaos and madness.

I began this work in many ways as a result of a feeling of boredom that permeated my experience as a theatre artist: I was bored of the vicious, incestuous and sterile cycle of theatre, where colleagues attend each other's shows, all dealing with well-known texts written by well-known playwrights, and having no connection to reality or to the actual

Z. Daccache, BA, MA, RDT (✉)
Catharsis – Lebanese Center for Drama Therapy, Mount-Lebanon, Lebanon
e-mail: zeina@catharsislcdt.org

© The Author(s) 2016
S. Pendzik et al. (eds.), *The Self in Performance*,
DOI 10.1057/978-1-137-53593-1_16

stories of everyday life. We all applauded but nothing changed. I began to question theatre artists and asked myself: Why have we isolated ourselves? Why were we performing only in front of the 'educated' while losing sight of the larger portion of society? Where were the actors? Where were the people who wanted to communicate something of vital importance to the audience? What about the immigrants we encounter daily on Beirut's streets, the addicts residing in the rehabilitation centers? What about the mentally ill patients forgotten in hospitals or the 7000 inmates crammed into the country's overcrowded prisons? I started to wonder what would happen if the artists on stage were drawn from the people who have something in their guts, something concrete and worthwhile to say, and motivated to put their hearts and souls into making change happen, would hold 'the mirror up to nature'? (*Hamlet*, Act 3, scene II).

I was also closely observing the way in which advocacy for certain populations' needs and rights was being conducted in Lebanon. I realized that it has always been accomplished via institutions or activists: We hear members of the Parliament or activists speaking up for prisoners' rights or see a nongovernmental organization conducting a campaign to stop domestic violence; but we never hear the message coming directly from the concerned population. We watch the TV news reporting of endless riots in prisons, or showing a woman crying in front of the camera as she tells how her husband beats her and her children. Some tears run down our faces, but five minutes later, we forget what we saw... perhaps, because, the message was delivered with too much anger or intensity and, therefore, is out of our comfort zone.

So, in 2006, I decided to see how theatre and drama therapy can live and grow in the most forgotten places and the most difficult situations. I felt that the resulting performances would need to be constructed from the actors' words, stories, experiences, reflections, hopes, dreams, and that by incorporating these sources into the plays, the performances could lead to real change. In a way I consider myself to have been an autodidact. At the time, I had no idea of the existence of terms such as *autobiographical*, *self-revelatory* and *auto-ethnographic* forms of *therapeutic theatre* (Emunah, 2015; Pendzik, 2013; Spry, 2001); and I admit I had not even researched them. I saw performances related to participants' real stories during my drama therapy studies at Kansas State University and in workshops, but felt these would not be the same methods I would be using one day. I did not even have a clear vision of the outcome of what my potential work might be; I just felt that it was worth trying and that the path would not be easy. Yet I believed that a performance enacted by prisoners in front of society at large (and not just staged for the 'educated elitist' audience), based on their own stories, could make a change: in them, in the society, and, ultimately, in the policies used against them. I felt that through their artistic product they could self-advocate, and thereby communicate their message to the decision-makers; this time, however, using a constructive means—the artistic product—rather than a bloody riot or a cheesy TV report.

In pursuit of this aim I integrated all I had learned from a life of study and training: in London, with Philippe Gaulier, for whom theatre was an emancipatory tool for anyone and everyone, and who taught his students that a 'boring actor', 'boring message' and 'boring performance' are the devil of theatre (Gaulier, 2008); and at Volterra Prison in Italy, where I had assisted Italian theatre director Armando Punzo, who later became a close colleague, training with me in Lebanese prisons. Punzo's staging of works by Shakespeare, Brecht, and Virgil, as well as other Italian playwrights, acted by the inmates both within and outside the walls of Volterra Prison and in front of large audiences, have become a feature of Italian theatrical life (Bernazza & Valentini, 1998; Punzo, 2013). My BA in Theatre Studies at Saint Joseph University in Beirut in 2000, my graduate studies in Psychology at Haigazian University in Beirut and in drama therapy at Kansas State University, and the training in drama therapy I undertook with drama therapists Armand Volkas, Sally Bailey and John Bergman (the three of whom later imparted workshops in collaboration with me in the Lebanese prisons), and Tobi Klein (among others), all opened my eyes to the understanding of group process, and taught me how the use of great drama therapy techniques can lead to a great performance.

So in 2007, in Lebanon, assisted by a grant from the European Union, I implemented a drama therapy project in the largest detention center for men in Lebanon: Roumieh Prison. My first task was to decide what kind of performance the project would lead to. Would I adapt a text? Write one? Adapt one from the inmates' own stories? Have each inmate's real story on stage enacted by himself? Create a new text with them from their collective experience? I had no clue or colleague near me, because I was (and to this day still am) the only drama therapist in Lebanon.

ROUMIEH PRISON

Roumieh Prison, the largest and most notorious Lebanese male prison, has around 3500 inmates residing in buildings that were primarily built to house a maximum of 1000. In fact, the squalid conditions of the prison have led to several riots against the administrators over the course of the prison's history. Criminals who had committed widely different crimes live inside the same small room (seven to ten persons in a room made for two). An inmate might be imprisoned for robbery and leave jail having mastered drug-dealing while inside. Racism and classism are also big issues in the institution: The poor are treated mostly as servants while the rich have more rights. Furthermore, few and rare are the actions that have been taken in Lebanon to reeducate or rehabilitate criminals. In addition, there is a strong need in Lebanon for the revision of laws related to the penal code, such as the abolition of the death penalty, the modification of the rules applicable to prison management, and the unfairness of being held without trial for a long time.

In 2007 the establishment of a drama therapy/theatre program inside Roumieh (or indeed inside any Lebanese prison) was an unprecedented act, as art, drama, or music programs have been only very rarely introduced into prisons. Therefore, after the European Union had approved the financing of the project, I still faced the challenge of explaining it to Lebanese government officials (who thought I was crazy to believe that theatre—a luxury, in their opinion—was necessary and useful in a prison). They repeatedly refused for a whole year, but I was stubborn and persisted. In February 2008, they finally approved the request to start the project, but still demanded that I ask for all kinds of approvals at each stage of the process.

The whole year of dealing with the bureaucracy was very useful to me, as I gained a glimpse of the frustration that inmates experience on a daily basis. I imagined how many demands and requests they needed to write in order to get a ten-minute visit from their children, or even to know when their next court hearing was taking place. I started to prepare the drama therapy sessions while I was still awaiting clearance. I read the penal code and realized that most of it had not been updated since the 1940s. I read about the riots that had taken place in the last ten years, the reasons for them, their outcomes.

In February 2008, the project began—a journey charged with challenging and unforgettable moments. The 15 month project included a four-month period of drama therapy sessions with different groups; then a play was to be prepared during a seven-month rehearsal period. The final result was to be performed for two months inside prison. 250 inmates responded to the initial call for the drama therapy sessions. Few had ever previously taken part in theatre or any kind of therapy, but they were excited about the chance to express themselves. Others were reluctant and doubtful about the project; they viewed us just like another group of people coming to sell them hope, but never achieving any goals.

Of the group that participated in the initial drama therapy sessions, some did not want to continue to the play production; others could not commit to the whole period, as their sentences were shorter than the length of the project, and some were moved to other prisons in accordance with the usual prison administration policies. All of this was accompanied by endless bureaucratic hurdles, and the difficulty of working in a prison led me to wonder if I would really be able to persevere and see the project through. In the end, 45 inmates participated in the theatre production, many of whom were facing the death penalty or a life sentence.

Slowly, the themes of the play began to emerge: the prejudice they endure from society, the injustice of the sentences issued with reference to an obsolete penal code that is older than their age, the long incarceration periods that began even before being sentenced, no reduction of sentences for good behavior, racism inside the prison, the unknown future, guilt towards one's self and towards the victim(s), coping with their family (if they had any).

Many inmates had great music or dance backgrounds. Different nationalities, and therefore, cultures and religions, were involved: Lebanese, Nigerians, Iraqis, Bangladeshis and Palestinians. Some inmates wanted to do monologues, others short scenes, others to express themselves through dance or music. Ultimately, I needed a larger structure around which to bring together all of these smaller performances. I decided to incorporate the pieces inside a Lebanese adaptation of *Twelve Angry Men*—the 1954 teleplay by American writer Reginald Rose.

Although in Lebanon there is no such judiciary system called a *jury* (only a judge issues the sentences), I found that the theme of prejudice can be best portrayed in this play—a play that follows a jury deliberating about the death sentence of an 18-year-old boy who has been accused of killing his father. In the play, 11 members of the jury are absolutely convinced that the suspect is guilty and refuse to reconsider the case, guided by deep prejudice and faulty judgments that nearly lead them to commit a miscarriage of justice. In our Roumieh adaptation, titled *12 Angry Lebanese*, the members of the jury were played by inmates, resulting in a reversal of roles. The inmates would play our role—the presumably objective society—judging and debating the fate of a suspect on trial. Roumieh represents a microcosm of Lebanon and the sectarian groups that form the national policy; thus, our adaptation also occasioned interaction and dialogue between these divergent sociopolitical constituencies. As the jury argues about the defendant's case, they become sidetracked by their own agendas, ignorance, and stereotyping. In that regard, the production not only portrayed the situation of the prisoners, but also reproduced the sociopolitical situation in Lebanon.

Indeed each actor/inmate brought his unique life experience to the adaptation. So instead of the European watchmaker, it was the Nigerian guy looking for work in Lebanon; instead of character number five, who grew up in a violent slum, it was the Palestinian refugee who grew up in the poor Palestinian camps in Lebanon. The performance was punctuated by monologues—personal testimonies that we carefully developed during the rehearsal period.

One monologue–a collage of many stories–was built up from weekly sessions that included only the group of inmates facing death penalties and life sentences. We worked through metaphors to express the long years of incarceration. Here is an excerpt:

> I am the Grandpa of the inmates. Why? Because I have been here for 18 years… 18 years is 216 months. It is 6570 days. It is 157,440 hours. It is 9,446,400 minutes. It is 566,784,000 seconds. But I'm not serving an 18-year sentence. I'm serving a life sentence. Life sentence is feeling sorry again and again for what you have done. Life sentence is listening to the 'new' inmates telling you they miss their wives, while yours has divorced you the day you entered prison… In your head everything remains the same…
> I was shocked when my mother told me last year that my cousin Sawsan, who was nine years old when I got imprisoned, got married… Mum! How could they marry a nine-year-old kid? Mum reminded me that Sawsan was 27 years old now!

Eight men spoke. I gathered all their thoughts in one monologue and one group member interpreted it. The guy was chosen by the group (rather than me); it was their stories, and therefore their casting too.

The musically inclined inmates had their weekly sessions to create a soundtrack for the play. They ended up being on stage the whole time, performing 12 songs during the show. These songs were written and composed by them, and revolved around themes agreed upon by the group:

> *Your Judgment burned me Dear Judge,*
> *I am in Prison and you're doing just fine;*
> *I'm building just like a free man.*
> *I'm building and learning how to become more criminal.*
> *It's out of the question that you forget me. You leave me detained and frozen.*
> *You neither judge nor forgive me… Your bird I am.*
> (Quote from the song Your Bird I Am, from the soundtrack of *12 Angry Lebanese*).

Others—great painters—wanted to do graffiti on the walls. Thus, along the peeling concrete of the walls, ran slogans in Arabic and English:

> *'War Makes Prisoners, Peace Hangs Them…'*
> *'I have always found that mercy bears richer fruits than strict justice*
> Abraham Lincoln'

Every day, the actors brought in monologues, texts, and songs they wanted to integrate into the performance. Many were scenes about suggestions for new laws. This process led us to consult activist lawyers and judges, in order to give their advice on what would be the best possible modifications the inmates could suggest in their play. Having read the penal code myself, I was impressed by a law called 'the reduction of sentences for good behavior' that was issued in 2002 but never implemented, and that even policy makers hardly remembered. I even met several times with the policy maker who has drafted the law in 2002 in order to try to understand the reasons for its non-implementation. He said there were no concrete reasons: it just went into oblivion. I also asked (and received) approval from members of the parliament to allow me to attend their weekly sessions in order to suggest certain amendments concerning prison policies. A new scene was born: one person played the judge, another, the inmate, demanding the reduction of his sentence, reminding the policy makers about his rights. Two months after the end of play, to which we had invited all policy makers (e.g., ministers, MPs in charge of the justice system), the Law for the Reduction of Sentences for Good Behavior began to be implemented.

Rateb, sentenced to seven years for rape, proposed a monologue repenting of his crime. Some of the other men threatened to leave the group if Rateb performed the piece. 'We can't work with a criminal,' they said. I couldn't believe it. 'Wow,' I replied, 'If that's the case, then I'm heading out, because I can't work with 45 criminals! Why don't you all quit? At least we will have one real scene with someone who would have benefited from drama therapy: Rateb.'

With inmates like Rateb, I worked often in individual sessions, applying psychodrama techniques like role reversal. For example, we played that he is the victim attending the play or he is someone among the audience hearing Rateb speak. As we did that, Rateb gained a lot in terms of developing a sense of empathy, and putting himself into another's shoes. Finally, when the group first heard Rateb's story, they called him 'Brother', and, later on, even the audience ended up offering him jobs upon his release, and chances for a better future.

At the end of the first project, Catharsis (the Lebanese Center for Drama Therapy that I had founded in 2007) received a continuous clearance from prison authorities for offering drama therapy in prisons. Such sessions became one of the components that influence an inmate's application for a reduction of sentence.

BAABDA PRISON

A few months after the end of the first project, the women inmates began to ask for this kind of work in their own prisons; and in 2011, drama therapy started at the Baabda prison for women. Drama therapy became a continuous activity inside both Roumieh and Baabda; and in 2012, with funding from the Swiss Foundation Drosos, the preparation for a new play started, this time enacted by the women inmates in Baabda Prison.

The women inmates lived in the same conditions as the men: overcrowded prisons, long detention periods, etc. However, their reasons for being behind bars were totally different: most of these women were there because of the patriarchal society in which we live. Nine out of the 25 who joined the drama therapy sessions had killed their husbands, as there was no law to protect them from domestic violence; six were there for adultery, which is regarded as a crime in Lebanon. (Although the law applies for both men and women, no man has ever been incarcerated for committing adultery.) The rest were there for drugs, stealing, etc. Early marriage was a common experience for almost 90 per cent of them. Some had been forced to marry at the age of 12 or 14. They had a deep desire to communicate their stories to the outside world, in order to make sense of the lives they had led. As one of them puts it, 'Perhaps our stories would serve to raise awareness to other girls outside, and who knows, maybe our play would help to finally generate laws to protect women ...'

I had no doubt this time about making a full play based on their personal stories. Their stories were deeper than any script I have read. No adaptation of a well-known text would work. We agreed together that the play would be a series of monologues, short scenes made by a maximum of two people, and perhaps a dance, and we decided to call the play *Scheherazade in Baabda*, referring to the legendary Arabic queen and the storyteller *of One Thousand and One Nights*, who told stories to Shahryar to save her life.

At that time Armand Volkas, my drama therapy teacher from San Francisco, visited Lebanon to impart alternative training workshops at Catharsis, and I invited him to facilitate two sessions at the women's prison in order to help with the production of the play. He facilitated a beautiful exercise with the women, in which each one had to think of an object that means a lot to her, one which she cherishes, and tell the story behind it. One woman told a story of adultery through a diary, another shared about her submissive life with her husband through a violin that he played. '*He had his hobbies... his violin... his own things... I never had anything that I could call mine...*'

Using the same technique as in Roumieh, the women were divided in groups: one group consisted of those who were forced into early marriage and ended up murdering their husbands; another group decided to present a flamenco dance, telling their common story as women in a patriarchal society through dance.

ETHICS

In both prisons attention to ethics was essential. Not all the inmates wanted to perform on stage; some did not want to do their own monologues, as they were afraid that the audience would point them out saying:

'Oh, she killed her husband…' In this sense, working in smaller groups was very helpful. For instance, each of the women who had murdered her husband told her story, reflected on it, and listened to the other inmates' stories, thus feeling less lonely in their suffering. In the end, when all the bits and pieces of the stories were dramaturgically embroidered into one text, the group chose one or two persons to say the text in front of the audience. So the monologue would hold the stories of nine women, as if it was a single story. It was made clear to the audience from the beginning of the show that the texts they are going to hear are a compilation of many stories blended as one. Another way of handling this ethical issue was to change the names in the play. Fadia became Nadia, Nisrine became Sonia. In those cases where the storyteller did not want to be on stage but did want to have her powerful story presented, written consent was requested from her to have someone else enact it (of course under a fictional name). I remember one woman who knew that her son who would be in the audience, and wouldn't accept her saying that finally, in prison, she feels at home, as she had never had a proper home outside. After discussing the matter in the group, it was decided she would not be on stage out of courtesy to the family member who thought she was the happiest mother on earth. Indeed, the effect of seeing her text on stage enacted by someone else was as cathartic for her and the audience as if she had enacted it herself, reminding me of the power of Playback Theatre.

DISCUSSION AND CONCLUSION

The women, just like the male inmates, showed their play for two months in 2012 inside prison to a wide audience of policy makers, media, their families, human rights activists, general public, etc.; and the award-winning documentaries depicting both experiences (*12 Angry Lebanese—The Documentary* and *Scheherazade's Diary*) toured the world, carrying the inmates' messages even farther. Finally, in April 2014, after a succession of publicized cases of domestic violence, years of Lebanese civil activism by many NGOs, and many screenings of the play *Scheherazade in Baabda* and of the documentary *Scheherazade's Diary*, a bill for the Protection of Women and Family Members from Domestic Violence was passed by the Lebanese Parliament.

Both of these experiences confirmed my belief that theatre and drama therapy can live in the most forgotten places, grow in the most difficult situations, and the resulting performances built around and written from the actors' own words, stories, experiences, reflections, hopes, and dreams, can lead to real change. Since the end of *Scheherazade*, I continued to offer drama therapy sessions in both prisons, developed a program for the mentally ill residing in Lebanese prisons and led drama therapy projects with other disadvantaged populations. In 2013, the play *From the Bottom of my Brain*, performed by the residents of Al Fanar hospital for neuro-psychiatric disorders, saw the light, conveying the sincere desire of actors/inmates to build a bridge that reconnects them to the world. In addition, in 2014 the play *Shebaik Lebaik* with migrant domestic workers (MDWs) was held under the High Patronage of the Minister of Labor, consisting of short scenes and monologues from their own stories and dances from the respective participating nationalities (Ethiopia, Senegal, etc.). MDWs in Lebanon are at risk of exploitation since they are excluded from the Lebanese labor law and subject to immigration rules based on employer-specific sponsorship, known as the Kafala system. The play offered suggestions of extending the coverage of the Lebanese labor law to domestic workers.

Looking back at the 12 years in which I have conducted drama therapy/theatre with marginalized populations, I am still unsure what label to give to the kind of theatre I do: I have done one adaptation of a well-known text in the first project (*Twelve Angry Men*), which could be called Therapeutic Theatre (Snow, D'Amico, & Tanguay, 2003), yet I am not sure if I will adapt again. A big part of my work consists of writing texts in collaboration with lawyers, inviting high patronage and attendance by ministers to each play, and attending and participating in parliamentary sessions myself; yet I am not sure if what I do should be called Legislative Theatre (Boal, 2005). Likewise, although most of the time the monologues included in the plays are a collage of different real stories composed by the group or the actual story of the teller, I am not sure if I'd call it ethnotheatre (Saldana, 2005), self-revelatory performance (Emunah, 2015), or autobiographical therapeutic performance (Pendzik, 2013). In a way, I don't really want to name it. Perhaps naming it will make me and the actors abide by a certain process or method, whereas I keep discovering through the group I work with what should be done, which method should be used, on a daily basis. Perhaps I would rather call it *Their Theatre*, as in the end their plays are performed in their spaces, using their capabilities, their words, their audience and their messages. Drama therapists and theatre directors are—and will always remain—in the role of facilitators, helping the populations they work with to convey their own messages and make the change they need to see happen, not the change we want to see happen.

I will end by quoting some words spoken by the women inmates at the end of every performance of *Scheherazade in Baabda*. These words differed from performance to performance. Depending on the feeling of the moment, each woman spoke a sentence to the audience.

> '*A man is born from a woman's womb.*'
> '*I won't differentiate anymore between my son and my daughter.*'
> '*Did you like me?*'
> '*I wish I was told "no" when I was younger.*'
> '*No more self-destroying mistakes.*'
> '*I want to be a woman again. I'm tired of playing the role of a man in my life.*'
> '*I won't look down anymore. I will hold my head high.*'
> '*If my son ever beats his wife, I would take her side, not his.*'
> '*I had never known freedom until I entered prison.*'
> '*I allowed my husband to cross limits.*'
> '*I wish we have met elsewhere.*'
> '*Visit us again!*'
> '*My fate can change… So history can change too.*'

REFERENCES

Boal, A. (2005). *Legislative theatre: Using performance to make politics.* London: Routledge.

Bernazza, L., & Valentini, V. (1998). *La compagnia della fortezza.* Catanzaro, Italy: Rubbettino Editore.

Emunah, R. (2015). Self-revelatory performance: A form of drama therapy and theatre. *Drama Therapy Review, 1*(1), 71–85.

Gaulier, P. (2008). *Le Gégèneur/The Tormentor.* Paris: Editions Filmko.

Pendzik, S. (2013). The poiesis and praxis of autobiographical therapeutic theatre. Unpublished manuscript of the Keynote Speech presented at the *13th Summer Academy of the German Association of Theatre-Therapy*, Remscheid, Germany.

Punzo, A. (2013). *E' ai vinti che va il suo amore. I primi venticinque anni di autoreclusione con la Compagnia della Fortezza di Volterra.* Firenze, Italy: Ed. Clichy.

Rose, R. (1954). *Twelve angry men (teleplay).* Westinghouse Studio One.

Saldana, J. (2005). *Ethnodrama: An anthology of reality theatre.* Walnut Creek, CA: AltaMira Press.

Snow, S., D'Amico, M., & Tanguay, D. (2003). Therapeutic theatre and well-being. *Arts in Psychotherapy, 30,* 73–82.

Spry, T. (2001). Performing autoethnography: An embodied methodological praxis. *Qualitative Inquiry, 7*(6), 706–732.

CHAPTER 17

Reflections on *terrorists of the heart*: A Couple's Performance on Loss and Acceptance

Jules Dorey Richmond and David Richmond

In light of autoethnography and healing, in this chapter we reflect on our collaborative, autobiographical performance duet, *terrorists of the heart*—braiding performance text, reflective writing, and theoretical contextualization. We have always been bemused by the statement, 'it's not personal, it's just business,' as everything is personal, processed via our senses. This is why we have always started our research explicitly from the personal. In *autobiographical performances*, memory is presented as personal narrative and the private is made public.

Academic and theorist Annette Kuhn's 'memory work' acts as a paradigm for connecting personal history to public event, and, as with all public autobiographical utterances, that question so eloquently phrased by Annette Kuhn needs to be addressed: 'what right have I to subordinate history to my own puny existence?' (2002, p. vii). The making of the work has to also deal

J.D. Richmond, BA, MFA, FHEA (✉) • D. Richmond, BA, MA, SFHEA
York St John University, York, UK
e-mail: J.DoreyRichmond@yorksj.ac.uk; d.richmond@yorksj.ac.uk

© The Author(s) 2016
S. Pendzik et al. (eds.), *The Self in Performance*,
DOI 10.1057/978-1-137-53593-1_17

241

with this inherent reactionary critique, raising the question: whose interests are being served by our silence, our forgetting, and our passivity?

We will investigate our *autoethnographic performance* work, *terrorists of the heart*, which looks at loss in the wake of parenthood and aging. The work also considers the wider cultural backdrop of socialism's unfulfilled promise and our dreams of living in a more equal, just, ecological and cooperative world.

In his influential essay, *Interventions and Radical Research*, American performance studies scholar Dwight Conquergood sets out a case, appropriating the French philosopher Michele de Certeau's pithy saying, 'What the map cuts up the story cuts across' to speak of different domains of knowledge 'to open the space between analysis and action, and to pull the pin on the binary opposition between theory and practice' (2002, p. 145). The form of this text will follow the trope of our arts practice influenced by Dwight Conquergood, which is to braid subjugated knowledge (*the story*) with legitimatized knowledge (*the map*), in this case the lived experience of our co-embedded lives, the co-emergent understanding of what it is we do and critical thinking around the political context we find ourselves in. We utilize *bricolage* as a coherent methodology bringing a constellation of ideas, practices, and images to bear on the work, as an approach to inquiry explicitly based on notions of eclecticism, emergence, flexibility, and plurality (Rogers, 2012).

We look at the audience as 'they' enter; 'they' and 'we' are in the same light, same space and same time, and so it begins.

Things to be outed: we have been married for 27 years; we are long-term collaborating artists having made ten original works together, whilst also working for theatre companies throughout the United Kingdom and Europe; we are parents to a daughter; and pedagogues in the same theatre program at York St John University, UK. We made the performance work, *terrorists of the heart*, after a ten-year break in our collaborative performance-making, during which we were busy with a different collaboration, that of co-parenting. Creating the time and space to work together was an important commitment to action, but what action? Aside from the desire to make a show we had no thoughts of content. We very quickly understood that we were not the same people we had been a decade earlier, when we had last collaborated on a duet; we had aged, our bodies had gotten fat, weak and stiff. Now in our living room studio we discovered we could no longer throw and carry each other as we had ten years prior; our knees were shot, our backs out of whack, our bellies in the way, and we found the physical aspect of our work was mainly helping each other up from the floor. We were confronted by the passing of time and the toll it had taken on our bodies, which unequivocally informed us that we were dealing with loss. We had let ourselves slip away without even realizing it.

Now, acutely aware of our physical failings and feelings of *loss* we consciously mined this territory further. We asked each other questions about loss, and we wrote the answers down.

> *We have words we are about to say out loud and they are on a clipboard next to us, they are the words we have written that we will speak.*

We discussed the fact that the great socialist future—the one where and when women and men were treated as equals; the color of your skin had no bearing on your prospects; the class divide had evaporated and no one lived in poverty; one's sexual orientation was of no note; and everyone was celebrated for what they could do, as opposed to being defined for what they could not—had remained a dream. We felt fully complicit in not bringing this (utopian) future to fruition—we had failed. Somewhere and somehow life had sneaked up on us.

It was at this point that we began to grieve: we grieved for the world-as-a-better-place, the one that we spoke about when we first met and were going to build together; we grieved for the people we were—young and in love and invincible together; and we grieved for the versions of ourselves that we had projected into the future, who never materialized. We discovered that we had quite a lot of grief and we did a lot of crying. We had to confront our biggest fear, that, perhaps, we no longer loved each other.

It was these concerns that led us to make the performance, *terrorists of the heart*. We only ever make work to try to understand the world we live in. German philosopher and cultural critic Walter Benjamin (1892–1940) reminds us of the positional nature of memory, of not just what is remembered but of the person who remembers, of the here and now in the there and then of memory.

As always, we followed Walter Benjamin's axiom in our thinking/ making.

> He who seeks to approach his own buried past must conduct himself like a man digging. Above all, he must not be afraid to return again and again to the same matter; to scatter it like one scatters earth, to turn it over as one turns over the soil. (In Jennings, 2005, p. 576)

As theatre makers we had no choice, but to keep digging, paying close attention to our grief. We wondered why, before the process of making this show together, we had not been aware of this sadness; though it was clear that the sadness had been there all along, we had not paid attention to it, or each other.

We look at you, we look at each other, we look at you and smile.

So we looked at ourselves, our life together, the world around us and started work. Chang defines autoethnographic performance as a research method that enables researchers to use data from their own life stories as situated in sociocultural contexts in order to gain an understanding of society through the unique lens of self (Chang, Ngunjiri & Hernandez, 2012, p. 18). In our research we looked for structures to hold us and, of course, the work, as in so many ways they are indissoluble. This is when we discovered Elisabeth Kübler-Ross' (1969) *Five Stages of Grief*: denial; anger; bargaining; depression; acceptance. So we used these five stages of grief to inform the making of the work and ultimately to structure the composition of the piece.

Denial

Jules: *... It didn't really touch me, it didn't really affect me, nothing can harm me, nothing gets to me, you can't hurt me, I am Teflon (nothing sticks), I didn't want the job, I like being on my own, I prefer my own company, I didn't really want to go, I will get better, I will be better...*

Jules puts on balaclava.
David pulls balaclava up

David: *it's not true, you are better than this, I am better than this, she is better than this, we are better than this, they are better than this...*

Anger

David: *I rage against those that lie*
Jules: *it was about this time that you began to accuse me of being angry*
David: *I rage against those that lie*
Jules: *I remember our rows*
David: *I rage against those that cheat*
Jules: *you taught me to shout*

Bargaining

David: *... I have made a Faustian pact, for the lives of my loved ones, for both of you.*

I will give my life for yours no matter what—no matter when. My only hope is that this bargain will be honored.

If I am prepared to give my life for yours it implies I am prepared to take a life for yours... For her... For you...

Jules: *A trade off... I'll do this, if you do that approach to life came late to me; I suppose it wasn't until I became a mother myself and my own time got severely pressed that I learned the need to bargain in order to buy myself some space and time to do nothing—and I mean, literally, nothing... as I don't remember being able to muse back then when I first became a mum ...*

Depression

David: *Feeling a bit low*

Feeling less than worthy, loving, kind, brave, clever. Spending so many, but maybe not many enough, hours crying.

I keep asking myself, Why go on?

Why try to keep it up?

Appearances, trousers, spirits, It all seems so pointless now

Jules: *My short-term memory depresses me—I walk into rooms and I don't know why I'm there, I meet people, there's a recognition, but for the life of me I don't know who they are. I can't remember names anymore or words for things. I'm frightened that one day I won't even recognize you*

Acceptance

David: *Average—in work—love—play*

I feel I can't change anything, that is of course what 'they' want,—but I know I can change everything. And if we do it together we can change the world, think of it, us in this room changing the world.

Who was the first person that sat in Tahrir Square in Cairo and said, 'I am not moving until it all changes'

Who was the first person in East Berlin on that fateful night—who shouted, 'We are the people'. We are the people.

David pulls the balaclava down

David stands, Lies down

Jules gets up & puts flowers by David

Jules sits down & pulls up balaclava

Jules: *saying yes when you want to scream no, that not everything will be done how and when I want... that this has nothing to do with me,*

*that I am not the center of the universe, that I haven't got a magic
wand or the power to make everything alright, it is just random that
this has happened.*

Going through these stages allowed us to work through our feelings and
locate ourselves in the present. We were middle-aged; the age where we
should make a will, which led us to make a show that became a living will.

Jules: *…give all my clothes to Grace—even though they will all be too small
          for her now
          Use up all my art materials to make art together
          Dance together at least once a week
          Spend Sunday mornings in bed with the papers
          Read to one another
          Brush and plait Grace's hair and remember the simple pleasure I got
          from this…*
David: *… when it is my time to die—I want the last touch to be yours
          I want to know I am dying and to be ready
          And for those that loved me and liked me at some point or another—
          to party on a beach and tell stories of my foolishness.*

This further enabled us to understand, to reconcile, the 'us' of then
and the 'us' of the ever-shifting ineffable now, as well as project into the
future a world in which we would be no longer. Once we understood that
we were in the territory of grief and loss we were able to situate ourselves
within the continuum of our lives/life and begin to take control. We talked
about a manifesto of love, a way of reconceiving the world we wanted to
live in—and this subsequently became the title of the work, until it met its
first audience. We put on our work clothes, for him black suit, black shirt,
black rubber clogs and balaclava; for her black blouse, black skirt, black
tights, black rubber clogs and balaclava. We braided our five stages of grief
with acts of resistance. We danced. Over time, our dancing transformed
to Morris Dancing, a traditional form of English vernacular street dance.
As the work developed this became allogenically infected by various compositional strategies, i.e. slowed down, speeded up, marked through, etc.

In the show we each sat in a chair, six foot apart, facing forward, both
with a side table. On his table a jam jar of wild flowers, on hers a family
picture, both with a glass of water. We sat facing forward, looking at the
audience. We have the words we are about to speak on clipboards, as we
have not had the time to learn them by heart. Later the clipboards are

retained to ensure that it is clear these words that are spoken are also written.

We sit, we roll back our balaclavas and we look at each other and we look at you and so it goes on

Our encountering of our autobiography can only really be of value if it offers the witness an opportunity of reflecting on his or her story.

What can be said, though, purposefully and without hesitation, is that, in the face of all the evidence presented here, there is nothing 'mere' about autobiographical performances. The majority are also much more than 'merely about the self'. Rather, they are performances of aspiration and possibility, creative acts that have the potential to contribute to ongoing cultural transformations. Looking at the past through the present we are urged to consider the future and what we might choose to make there. (Heddon, 2002, p. 172)

The private/public problematic is exposed one step further when the personal narratives being played out are by a couple, where the lives lived together are longer than the lives lived apart. The longevity, proximity and the daily life of our co-embeddedness rendered us blind to each other, which the making and performing of *terrorists* countered by providing us individually and collectively with a reflective surface to see each other in the here and now. By opening our personal archive we ask—is it, perhaps, only in the drift and disturbance of time and the volatility of memory that we see who we were, who we wanted to be, and who we are now (not).

After the public showing/sharing, a structured conversation was facilitated using Liz Lerman's *Critical Response Process* (Lerman & Borstel, 2003)—a feedback system designed to facilitate an understanding of what artists have created by providing a structured dialogue between the audience and the performer, which aims to present practical pathways for developing the work further. The process follows four clear steps: (1) The audience tells the artist what in the work made an impact/has meaning for them; (2) The artist is given an opportunity to ask the audience questions about what they have presented; (3) The audience is given an opportunity to ask the artist questions; (4) Audience members are invited to address a particular aspect of the work, using the phrase, 'I have an opinion about… do you want to hear it?' The artist can accept or decline. Throughout this guided process the audience is instructed to use expansive vocabulary in order to communicate thoughts and feelings fully. We found this to be an extremely useful process in understanding and developing our material and we made several discoveries. It was clear we had something to say about aging, embedded, familial lives, which communicated to an audience beyond ourselves. The political material we had created needed to be pushed further to resist the possibility of it being read as irony, rather than the authentic belief that we needed to change how the world operates on us all. The scenographic elements needed to be thought through more coherently. Audience members' comments that we were like 'terrorists of the heart' led us to a more apt title for the show.

Performing in front of a critically friendly audience afforded us a fresh understanding of the performance itself, enabling us as writers, directors, and performers of our own stories an opportunity to deepen our understanding of what we had made, and not, necessarily, what we thought we had made. Through this new perspective we were able to re-draft and re-frame the performance material with greater clarity and objectivity. The testing out of performance material in front of an invited audience is a crucial stage of any devising process; after all, theatre is an art form that requires an audience to complete it.

So we reflected on some of the questions and observations made by the audience of friendly critics. The most significant aspect of feedback that we received was that the political list of demands, our manifesto of love, which we delivered towards the end of the piece, needed further consideration. Interestingly, no one in the critical feedback session offered an opinion about how to develop this material, and initially we did not know what to do; however, looking at our script we identified various compositional structures. We noticed we often used a kind of doubling; obviously there were two of us, offering two takes, and sometimes material was repeated but altered. For instance, in the *acceptance* section there is a litany of things that begin with the phrase, 'I'll never...' which later we repeat without this prefix, transforming our perspective on our situation by taking agency over our lives.

> Jules: ... *I'll never have a one-night stand*
> David: *I'll never be in a Mike Leigh film*
> Jules: *I will never die my hair green*
>   *Paint my room black*
>   *Have another baby*
> David: *I'll never make love one more time*

Subsequently becomes

Jules:	... *have a one night stand*
David:	*be in a Mike Leigh film*
Jules:	*die your hair green*
	Paint your room black
	Have another baby
David:	*make love one more time*

These clues helped us see that we could deliver our manifesto of love twice, and we decided to bracket the show with these demands. As a performance strategy we were asking the audience to re-look at this material, in light of the material that had gone before and after the initial iteration, in order to see what had changed. We were asking ourselves to look at ourselves, and asking the witness, in this discursive space, to look again at their own selves.

When we first presented the manifesto of love (our political demands) we performed it with sincerity but were dismayed to hear that our audience found it amusing. It was important for us that the material be received in the way we intended. So counter-intuitively, we decided to adopt a crude, almost comical delivery at the start of the show, to deliberately set ourselves up as naïve performers. The result was much hilarity, allowing us all to be in the same space at the same time with all of our collective vulnerabilities. Of course, what followed was highly personal material, concerned with loss in the wake of parenthood and aging, which the telling of now functioned as a rite of passage enabling an impassioned delivery of our manifesto of love towards the end of the show.

The positioning of our manifesto at the beginning and end of the performance gave us permission, for the second iteration of the manifesto, to discard the balaclavas—rendering us exposed, which had efficacy because the audience had witnessed through the performance the personal within the political discourse. Therefore the audience/performer relationship operated as a crucible for socially engaged mutuality, an understanding not only of what was being said, but also of the lives and motivation behind the text, asking the witnesses to reflect on their lives. In this way the work went beyond the making and performing of a theatre show, as the autobiographical aspects of *terrorists of the heart* and its functioning as a living will was explicit. The work was a genuine call to the audience/witness to re-look at their dreams for the future, to examine what they have let go, lost and may wish to reclaim, and to bear testimony to their own lives. This would not have been possible without an understanding of the political discourse inherent within the manifesto of love, and the wider loss in our collective culture.

Between 2010 and 2013 we performed *terrorists* on half a dozen occasions and with each performance we were acutely aware of our shifting perspectives towards the material. As time passed, most critically towards the end of the three-year period, we were aware that another gap of experience and understanding had opened up between our 'scripted selves' and the 'selves performing' the show, which echoed our initial realizations 'that we were not the same people.' Deidre Heddon (2002) problematizes this dissonance further when she says, 'The performer may perform the self, but one can never be entirely sure of who the self that is being performed is, nor in fact who the performer is, as both selves keep slipping' (p. 6).

These two distinct perspectives, the past and the future, generate a dissonance, of what Heddon (2008) refers to as a gap between the I/ we who is telling the story and the I/we who the story is about. Equally, there is a gap between the we who is telling the story and the we who witness the story and in some sense have to tell their story, if only to themselves, as Shoshanna Felman suggests, 'Through the bond of reading… the story of the Other…, as our own' (2003, p. 14).

We talk of loss, we talk of those times when we suffered, and we talk of those times when we were full of outrageous joy, and so it goes on.

Suzi Gablik articulates, in the *Re-enchantment of Art*, that there is an opportunity to re-animate and re-vitalize postmodern culture through a move away from patriarchal structures with its emphasis on separation and detachment, towards the feminine with emphasis on connectedness—participative, empathetic and relational modalities of engagement. Gablik asserts that 'the next historical and evolutionary stage of consciousness, in which the capacity to be compassionate will be central not only to our ideals of success, but also to the recovery of both a meaningful society and a meaningful art' (1995, p. 182).

We use compassion as a central tenet of our praxis and in *terrorists of the heart* we articulate both a personal and a political loss, which we attempt to come to terms with by contemplating and playing out our worst-case scenario—death of the other and living without them. Here the we is obliterated as each is rendered an I and not-I as we imagine life without the other and death. It is through this symbolic act, of dying in performance, that we are then enabled to metaphorically heal, as we come to terms with the people we have become in a renewed awareness of life as a continuous process of becoming and, through this, we take power by creating and performing a living will and by envisioning and calling for a more compassionate and just society.

Dance the Morris Political manifesto of love

David: *if we are going to move on from this it will have to be different; this is our political manifesto of love*

Jules: *these are our demands*

David: *no one can earn over £100,000 a year*

Jules: *banks, railways, land, the post office, shipping, buses are all state owned*

David: *women and men have equal pay, and home careers are paid the minimum wage by the state*

Jules: *the state is decentralised—local arrangements are made regarding producing and consuming food, excess is used for barter.*

David: *each arrondissement has its own forest and grows its own wood for fuel, all houses have solar panels and wind turbines, land can no longer be owned*

Jules: *the royal family are just the Windsors and have to work for a living, all their assets go to the state and all the palaces become homes for the elderly, poor and those most in need,*

David: *Albion becomes a republic of self-sufficient artisans*

Jules: *all young men at the age of 15 work on a maternity ward for a month.*

David: *all citizens of the free republic of Albion at the age of 18 engage in 2 years citizens' service—building houses, canals, hill farming, caring for the vulnerable, and engaging in international development and emergency rescue. And after the 2 years get 3 years higher education free.*

Jules: *Anyone wanting to become a citizen of Albion has to learn to cook the national dish....curry, and like um ..... Marmite and dance the mystery of the Morris.*

David: *there will be no religious schools; all religious education can take place Friday night, Saturday morning and or Sunday morning.*

Jules: *all children will be free-range and learn to be.*

David: *from cradle to grave*

Jules: *from cradle to grave*

David: *any commodity sold on the basis of sex will be banned—which is every-thing—but especially pornography and chocolate.*
Jules: *sex shall be celebrated but never sold*
David: *no longer the accumulation of excess*
Jules: *we will be born free and we will live and die free.*
David: *vote for love*
Jules: *vote for love*
J & d: *vote for love*
        J & D Kiss

'Sometimes family secrets are so deeply buried that they elude the conscious awareness even of those most closely involved' (Kuhn, 2002, p. 2). The work we made allowed us to access that everyday elusiveness, to bring to our conscious awareness the secret of our individual and collective loss. We started to talk to each other and we realised we were both living loss in such a profound way. Through the creative act of working together, sharing stories and by being vulnerable to each other, the carapace we had both built to protect ourselves from this elusive loss was ruptured; we allowed each other in, as when we first met—we shared stories to get to know each other (again). We did as Benjamin insists; we had 'to turn it as one turns the soil' (in Jennings, 2005, p. 576). The work became a re-investment and a re-affirmation of who we are as individuals and as a couple, bringing us back to ourselves and to each other, and our individual and collective engagement with politics, love, art and life.

The revelation of making, performing, and reflecting on the show is the fact that we love each other, still. It was this public iteration that prompted an audience member to refer to us as 'terrorists of the heart'.

We dance, we die, we talk, and we really mean the manifesto of love, so it goes on.

References

Chang, H., Ngunjiri, F. W., & Hernandez, K. C. (2012). *Collaborative autoethnography.* California: Left Coast Press.

Conquergood, D. (2002). Interventions and radical research. *The Drama Review, 46*(2), 112–130.

Felman, S. (2003). *What does a woman want? Reading and sexual difference.* London: Johns Hopkins University Press.

Gablik, S. (1995). *The re-enchantment of art.* New York: Thames and Hudson.

Heddon, D. (2002). Performing the self. *M/C: A Journal of Media and Culture, 5,* 5. http://www.media-culture.org.au/mc/0210/Heddon.html (01/10/2012).

Heddon, D. (2008). *Autobiography and performance.* Basingstoke and New York: Palgrave Macmillan.

Jennings, W. (2005). *Walter Benjamin: 1931–1934 vol. 2: Selected Writings.* Cambridge: Harvard University Press.

Kübler-Ross, E. (1969). *On death and dying.* New York: Scribner Press.

Kuhn, A. (2002). *Family secrets: Acts of memory and imagination.* London and New York: Verso.

Lerman, L., & Borstel, J. (2003). *Critical response process: A method for getting critical feedback on anything you make from dance to dessert.* London: Dance Exchange.

Rogers, M. (2012). Contextualizing theories and practices of bricolage research. *The Qualitative Report, 17*(7), 7–17.

CHAPTER 18

The Play as Client: An Experiment in Autobiographical Therapeutic Theatre

Maria Hodermarska, Prentiss Benjamin, and Stephanie Omens

This chapter defines and builds an argument for the concept of the *play as client* in the creation and performance of *autobiographical therapeutic theatre*. Drawing upon the experiences of the authors, all drama therapists, who were source, director, and actor of a single research project using a therapeutic theater process, the chapter considers how the play as client establishes aesthetic distance and contributes to the discourse on therapeutic and self-revelatory theater. The authors explore the ethical perspectives of this concept. By demonstrating the parallel process between caring for the play and caring for the human client, the authors examine the function of the drama therapist as a theater maker.

On The Floor by American playwright Cusi Cram (2013),[1] is a solo, ten-minute one-act play about Izzie, a pain-riddled, middle-aged college professor. It takes place at a colleague's dinner party at which Izzie is being fixed up with an academic named Hugo. When the play begins, Izzie has sought refuge in the bathroom, where she lies face down, toilet

M. Hodermarska, MA, RDT-BCT, CASAC, LCAT (✉) • P. Benjamin, MA
New York University, New York, NY, USA
e-mail: mh51@nyu.edu

S. Omens, LCAT (NY) MA-RDT, CCLS
Hackensack University Medical Center, Hackensack, NJ, USA

© The Author(s) 2016
S. Pendzik et al. (eds.), *The Self in Performance*,
DOI 10.1057/978-1-137-53593-1_18

bowl at her head, a purse full of pain pills just out of reach. In the opening moments, Izzie struggles for her handbag, winces in pain, rests, hums a few bars of *Suffragette City*, and then tries again. She fails a second time, and eventually gives up. The play is a comedy.

Not unlike Beckett's (1961) Winnie, who, despite being buried up to her waist in a mound of earth, exclaims that it is yet 'another happy day' (p. 23), Izzie faces her predicament brightly. She takes the audience into her confidence, like a trusted friend or therapist, as she contrasts the physical tolls of middle age—'knees puffy and tender,' spine 'uncertain and fragile' (p. 4)—with the thrill of her 'positively acrobatic' (p. 1) youth. She ruminates on the glories of sex and drugs and the scarcity of bidets in Manhattan. She makes up her face and takes her pills. Eventually, at play's end, she rises from floor to feet, and steps back into the waiting world.

On The Floor (Cram, 2013) is based on material that came from experiences of a drama therapy professor and clinician, the *source* (MH). The playwright, Cusi Cram, fictionalized them. The actor (SO) was a friend and colleague of the source and an experienced drama therapy clinician and supervisor. The director (PB) was a drama therapy student with many years' experience as a theater artist. The play was performed as part of the NYU Drama Therapy performance research series in therapeutic theater, *As Performance,* in an evening of short plays on the theme of the fading body. Dave Mowers, Executive Director of the series, offered all participants in this process his view that in therapeutic theater, the play, itself, is the client and asked, 'What are the implications ethical and otherwise of that concept?' (D. Mowers, personal communication, February 13, 2013). In this chapter, we take up Mowers' challenge and use it to explore the experiences of three individuals who were the source, director and actor, respectively, in this single therapeutic theater process.

THE PROJECT

It began humbly as a performative inquiry (Pelias, 2008), a form of duo-ethnography (Sawyer & Norris, 2013) or *co-researched autoethnography* (Bochner & Ellis, 2006; Ellis, 2007; Ellis & Bochner, 2000; Pelias, 2008)—researchers co-researching their own lived experience (in which the lived experience is the artifact studied)—through the creation of a theatrical fiction, a representational artifact of the lived experience. The product, the play, would be public. It was also an inquiry in therapeutic practice—how we hold stories, ours and each other's—when there are shared trajectories and points of identification.

By consciously engaging with those relational dynamics, we hoped to gain insight into how similar dynamics emerge in therapy, in certain forms of participatory action research, and in smaller fields like drama therapy, where dual relationships abound out of necessity. This experiment was praxis in ethics.

In psychodynamic terms, we were engaging intersubjective processes between and among us, confounding and disrupting the 'doer and done to' binary (Benjamin, 2004). In terms of power and privilege, we were investigating *intersectionality* (Crenshaw, 2004), understood as the inter-relationships between social divisions and identifiers, through the inversion or subversion of traditional power relationships: teacher to student, experienced clinical supervisor to emerging professional, and friend as psychodramatic double for friend. In theater terms, we were a company of co-creators.

Our research frame was the opposite of the one employed by qualitative researcher Carolyn Ellis and her colleagues (Ellis, Keisinger, & Tillmann-Healy, 1997). We did not process together during the experience as a full group. This decision was driven in part by the guerrilla nature of the project in which the director had eight weeks from beginning to end to present a finished work. Rather than extensive discussion and rumination about the experience as it was unfolding, we entered the project assuming that we all identified with Izzie's experience and that bringing her to life would therefore be rich and complex for everyone. Like Jonathan Fox's (1999) concept of *deep story* in Playback Theater, the risks here would be shared and palpable (pp. 1–2).

Our research interest concerned how we might do something therapeutic with a play that explored shared lived experience and the value for us as drama therapists in doing so. The subject matter was our story. We three were engaged in a commerce of shared truths about youth, womanhood, and the body, and the fictions we create and manipulate to protect ourselves from awareness of our own mendacity.

Along with shielding fictions, we built other safeguards into the process. The storyteller never saw the script. The actor only saw the script and didn't discuss the story with the source. The storyteller and the director knew what was true and the playwright and director knew what was fiction. The director, like a therapist, held the stories and brought them to life in the psychologically rich *empty space* (Brook, 1996) that is both the theater and therapy. The audience didn't know the source nor how much of the play was fictional and how much was factual. For the audience, it was just a play about the fading body of midlife and the corresponding *embodied presence* (Johnson, 2009) that comes, hopefully, with maturity.

A play can be a coalescing force, countering dissociation (Thomson & Jaque, 2011). It also acts as a boundary marker (Meldrum, 1999), providing the framework upon which narratives are arranged. In this way the play functions as a projective device, allowing the participants to safely engage, disguised yet differentiated. In our process, the play was the sacred object. Because externalized narrative 'allows us to separate story from self' (Cozolino, 2010, p. 171), the source, director, and actor could be both seen and unseen, understood yet protected.

On The Floor belonged to each of us and encapsulated our experiences. This mediation on self-experience shifted our understanding of the role dynamics we were inquiring about. We had stepped out of Benjamin's (2004) traditional therapeutic binary but remained in the dramatic world-view in which we began to see the play as the subject or object of care—the client—to which ethical duties of respect, competence and professional relationship are owed. In short, the play was the client, simultaneously the location of the therapy and the object of our care and ethical duty. It was our shared surrogate that allowed each of us to stand before the audience and tell a story that would be truthful to some extent for each of us about our own experience. Furthermore, conceiving of the play as client returned value and meaning and an *ethic of care* (Gilligan, 1982) to the aesthetic product of our work, not just its human process.

Ethics and Aesthetics in Therapeutic Theatre

Therapeutic theatre asks us to become more attentive to the art of the therapy. In drama therapy, axiological or values-based tensions are always present. These tensions exist in the dialectic between aesthetics (values relating to perception, sensation, experience) and ethics (values relating to actions taken or not taken); clinically, we operate at the nexus of the two. Ethics are at the heart of any therapeutic practice. Ethics are the standards we use to ensure a restraint from harm for our clients; these standards also remind us how we should act (Ridout, 2009). As drama therapists we embody and enact our ethics. Nowhere is this more vivid and risky than in the making of therapeutic theatre (Hodermarska, Landy, Dintino, Mowers, & Sajnani, 2015).

Drama therapy is a series of aesthetic choices but we rarely, as clinicians, conceive of them as such. We often focus on their ethical and clinical dimensions—the promotion of expression, aesthetic distance, insight, reciprocity, mutuality, and a sense of safety. Sajnani's (2012) concept of *relational aesthetics* in drama therapeutic praxis is the beginning of a necessary exploration into the relationship between the ethical dimensions of therapy and the aesthetic demands of the dramatic art form through which it occurs.

All therapy is, in part, a drama between client and therapist. Therapeutic theater can be seen as a conscious staging of the drama. In performance, the therapeutic relationship becomes heightened with everyone enacting the aesthetic risks of theater and the ethical risks of therapy. Client and therapist, student and teacher, performer and observer, actor and character become vulnerable subjects of study by the audience that can judge both the aesthetics and the ethics of the process (Kilgannon, 2014). As co-researchers in *On The Floor* we entered into and interrogated these binaries. We were able to do so by conceiving of the play as our shared client, and our responsibility to that shared client as our ethical and aesthetic obligation.

Our structure permitted each of us take risks as subjects, therapists, and artists, while being carried by the playwright's narrative imagination. There was twofold safety: the reflexivity and mutuality of the process (Ellis, 2007) decreased the potential for intrusion and harm, and the aesthetic distance (Landy, 1993; Scheff, 1979) of the fictionalized drama left us room to conceal what we chose. We could reflect upon our own experience and imagine the experiences of each other—two consummate therapeutic and dramatic actions. In life, fictions help us avoid the truth; in theater they are the lie that reveals the truth (Hodermarska, 2009; Emunah, 1994) that potentially leads to self-revelation.

For us, self-revelation was a by-product but not an intention. This distinguishes our process from drama therapist Renèe Emunah's (1994, 2009, 2015) form, *self-revelatory performance* (Self-Rev). In our process, the text, Moreno and Moreno's (1969) *cultural conserve*, was principal. The audience saw a play, rather than a theatrical piece depicting a psychological and drama therapeutic working through of the performer's personal issues, as in Self-Rev. The audience witnessed neither fact nor truth (Ridout, 2009) but an as-if or true-enough event that could potentially reveal their own individual truths.

As therapists performing therapeutic theatre we are always conscious of our relationship to each other and to the audience. For theater director

Peter Brook (1996) these axiological considerations are the foundation of working in the potential space that is the theater: in rehearsal the primary interpersonal relationship is between the actor/subject/director and in performance between the actor/subject/audience (1996, p. 100). The play is the fulcrum of the triangulated relationship, the form and structure for interaction and the place where all parties locate or avoid their truths. This process occurs both in reality and in the surplus reality, '... the reality beyond everyday reality, which is not visible, but very real' (Z. Moreno in Yalom, 2004, *The Double Life and Surplus Reality*, para. 2).

The structure of our process permitted us to honor the emergent surplus reality. The structure respected the inherent therapeutic action 'to tell' and the equal ethical obligation at times as client, therapist, artist, and audience to 'not tell' (Thompson, 2009a).

PERSONAL AND CO-CREATED SUBJECTIVITY IN AUTOBIOGRAPHICAL THERAPEUTIC THEATRE PROCESS

The anthropologist Barbara Rogoff (2003) noted how language and storytelling processes not only link individuals across time and over generations but also act as connective tissue, the subjective material that shapes cultural community.

In mapping both our subjectivities and intersubjectivities here, we hope to demonstrate how the performance of the play offered a metamorphosing of individual 'character and capacity' (Solnit, 2013, p. 11) and a deepening of community for and between each of us. What follows are our personal accounts of our experiences of subjectivity in the creation and performance of the play.

The Subjective Experience of the Source

As a practicing drama therapist, I (MH) have always been interested in how our humanity both promotes the most meaningful therapeutic movement [for and with a client] and, at other times, actually inhibits it. In 12-Step recovery programs, this paradox is articulated more bluntly in the slogan, 'We are only as sick as our secrets.' As therapists, when our own stories collide with, or even gently brush up against, those of our clients (or students, or friends), what is the mechanism that permits us to stay in those deep, hungry abysses and co-create from them?

My stories that I shared with PB were some not uncommon reminiscences of a maenad-like youth that included elements of the proverbial wild abandon—nightclub and after-hours scenes, substance use, and poor choices. Additionally, there were stories about the vicissitudes of mid-life. I always understood that whatever shame I held around my behavior in the past did not make me unique but, ironically, fairly ordinary, although this awareness did not keep me from feeling self-recrimination over the years. Nor did it prevent me from having to fight hard for compassion at times when my clients' stories mirrored my own (Hodermarska, 2009).

I trusted our ability to hold each other within, outside of, and alongside of the power positions of teacher/student and friend/friend because I trust the basic psychodramatic processes of doubling and role reversal (Moreno & Moreno, 1969). Any role reversal inevitably reveals the places of identification and shared experience. This is the basis of my praxis and my life.

As I age, I become increasingly aware of how my defenses are insufficient psychic protectors. Opacity is illusory. The truth is that I can be read. I am being read all the time, just as I am constantly reading others.

The play both revealed me and kept me well-hidden. No one in the audience at the time knew that I provided the source material for the play. As a drama therapist I firmly believe that fiction and metaphor can reveal and relate the truth more truthfully, and that fiction has the power to transform truth by locating deeper, ineffable meanings.

The Subjective Experience of the Director

I (PB) was attuned to the potential precariousness of the situation, particularly with regard to overlapping relationships—personal/professional, teacher/student, and actress/therapist. I was conscious of being the student, the novice whose work would be seen by the NYU drama therapy community. Would I be good enough? Would my collaborators, professors and experienced clinicians, be pleased? Who was I responsible to?

MH had given me permission to use the material in any way that I chose. We did not discuss its content or meaning. I pulled out themes and images that resonated, the first of these being lying on the bathroom floor. When I met with the playwright, stories converged, transforming MH's material into a co-shared narrative. Cusi was responsible for creating the play through which we could attach and orient ourselves. Her distanced eye provided us with a text with its own discrete identity. Script in hand, I as director had purpose and orientation.

My first responsibility was establishing safety. In rehearsing with SO, we focused on building trust so that she could fully inhabit and explore the role. I had to feel safe too. Initially, I was afraid of being alone in the room with her. Would she, as a drama therapist, find me out? Would she realize that I didn't know what I was doing? That I was a fraud? I noticed how those feelings echoed fears of being with clients in session, and with directors in rehearsal rooms. What ugly truths would they see?

I knew that SO felt similarly (she was bold and generous in voicing her insecurities). Our response to this anxiety was to progress tentatively, then more boldly, just as Izzie does in the play. In doing so, our working relationship developed. We traded stories about desire, pain, insecurity, and especially motherhood (poignant in retrospect, as I was pregnant but didn't yet know it), always in the context of the play. I recognized, perhaps more fully than in any other theatrical experience, that it was the play that we were serving. It was our client, needing our attention, patience, and care.

The Subjective Experience of the Actor

'I'm not an actor. OK, I was once, long ago, but this role no longer fits.' These were my words when I (SO) was originally approached to act in this play. I was haunted by the ghost of actor's-insecurity-past: 'Why do you want me?'

I agreed to be in this play primarily because of my relationship with the source. I was honored to render the playwright's version of her tale. So, despite my fears, I agreed to do it. Regarding the play as the client gave me the distance I needed to engage in the process. In my clinical practice, I am in service of the goals and needs of my clients.

I gave my fears to Prentiss to care for, trusting her, and I found my vulnerability easing. I soon began to know she would not criticize me, which allowed me to be far less inhibited 'on the floor' than I was able to be in my wild 20s, which was striking to me. I am a middle-aged woman now but I felt freer than my younger self.

THE PLAY AS CLIENT

The Experience of the Source

I would wait until the dress rehearsal to see how much of my real story remained in the play. When I finally saw the play, I experienced catharsis for the first time in my life as an audience member. It was a revelation. I was, in that moment, in the deepest existential sense, not alone.

The play held my cherished friendship of many years and it held my dear student and me in a space where we could honor the deeper meaning of care in our work. Everyone loved Izzie. No one saw her as shameful or damaged. I no longer needed to either.

'The play's the thing' (*Hamlet*, Act II, scene ii) (Jenkyns, 1996) that held me [and that I held] like I hold the people in my care. I was at once seen and hidden, protected by the aesthetic distance built into the process—masked and finally, gratefully, unmasked. This is precisely the process of intimacy and co-creation in treatment.

I confess: I had a reckless youth. I made poor decisions that I will forever regret. I put my body in danger. I did things that were unkind and disrespectful to myself and to others. Why confess here? Hamlet was correct. The play held my conscience and, furthermore, like a client, engaged me in the therapeutic arc that I experience in my most meaningful clinical processes when my truth is, to some extent, revealed alongside my client's and we meet in our human landscape.

The Experience of the Director

On The Floor, like every play, demanded that we take a point of view and deliver it with clarity. Specificity and discipline became paramount. In the rehearsal room we asked ourselves: Who is this woman? Where is she? Why? What is her relationship to the floor? To the world outside the door? To her physical and emotional pain and to all the 'stuff' she carries around with her: her purse, pills, lipstick? With a willingness to be unsure, attending to these questions with SO was where the work, and play, resided.

It wasn't until I saw the play in performance that I realized how much of myself was in Izzie. My own 'mottled parts' (Cram, 2013, p. 4)—those parts of myself that I try to keep hidden—from teachers, therapists, clients, husband, and now son—were on display. There I was: the slob, the narcissist, the victim, the slut. In my relatively anonymous role of director I could luxuriate in that recognition. But in the viewing it became clear that this was a shared recognition. The story did not belong to me, or the source, or the actress. The audience's presence brought it fully to life and allowed a therapeutic exchange to take place. For me, conceiving of the play as client amplified this resonance.

Play as Client: The Experience of the Actor

Approaching the play as the client afforded me clinical and aesthetic distance (Landy, 1993) from the role of Izzie. I was able to navigate the underbelly of the role without shame. Izzie was a role, my role, but Izzie was not me. In clinical practice, examining intersubjectivities and countertransferences requires me to face my self and my experience, and sometimes, my shame, directly. Studying Izzie's dark recesses, without being pulled down under with her, was thrilling. I could smell the musty fumes and dank waste of humanity and know it as part of me, yet not part of me.

I approached the play as client with the empathy I bring into the treatment room. The play/client required my embodied attention and reminded me of those embodied obligations to the client in the therapeutic space. The client in treatment has a layered history. I look for the clues in the history to support and help the client in their treatment. Just like the client, the play has a history to be unraveled: The character has a backstory and subtexts to be ascertained. Like treatment, the play occurs within a prescribed time frame from rehearsal to performance; and termination requires attention and care. My actress self was able to take more time with this client than I am often able to take in my clinical practice. As the actress, I could focus line by line, indulging in and savoring the metaphor I am always acting for my client, 'for real' as Emunah (1994) wrote. But this process returned me to the artist in me. I was acting for my role and for the play and in doing so acting for art, for the joy of pretend (and not.)

RECOMMENDATIONS FOR FURTHER STUDY AND CONCLUSION

We found that conceiving of the play as client in therapeutic theatre enhanced the intended therapeutic process. We appreciated the values of play making:

- From the perspective of the source of the play, having the experience authentically distilled, universalized, and given language by the writer.
- From the perspective of the director, specifying and fleshing out the play, finding its rhythm, beats, moments of breath and humor.
- From the perspective of the actor, honoring, identifying with, portraying with accuracy.

As drama therapists we are constantly moving between each of these theater-making functions in our therapeutic activities.

Many who study applied theatre practices, including Mary La France (2013) and James Thompson (2009a, 2009b), express concerns regarding the lack of thought to ethical practice in theater making. Regarding the play as the client is one way to frame a devised theater-making process that brings attention to the human vulnerabilities involved.

In this chapter we have addressed how conceiving of the play as the client afforded each of us opportunities on the continuum of emotion and distance for insight and catharsis throughout the process. The play itself was the therapeutic vehicle and therapeutic subject of our work.

The performance research process was imperfect and suffered from the uncertainties and shortcomings of what was really an exploration rather than a working within a recognized framework. We all understood that the notion of play as client has its limitations but in a situation in which there was no designated human client, we found it valuable in helping us stay mindful of professional duty and ethics.

The play as client brought three drama therapists, who regularly bring experience as actors to clinical practice, back full circle to the stage. In the process of caring for the play, we were, each of us, performing and being performed. In the process of caring for the play we were reminded as drama therapists that, '... at every instant the practical question is an artistic one...' (Brook, 1996, p. 98).

NOTE

1. The text of the play and footage of the performance of *On the Floor* can be found at: http://steinhardt.nyu.edu/scmsAdmin/media/users/cl1097/Onthefloor.pdf and http://steinhardt.nyu.edu/music/dramatherapy/photos/floor.

REFERENCES

Beckett, S. (1961). *Happy days.* New York: Grove.

Benjamin, J. (2004). Beyond doer and done to: An intersubjective view of thirdness. *Psychoanalytic Quarterly, 73*(1), 5–46.

Bochner, A. P., & Ellis, C. (2006). Communication as autoethnography. In G. Shepherd, J. S. John, & T. Striphas (Eds.), *Communication as perspectives on theory* (pp. 110–122). Thousand Oaks, CA: Sage.

Brook, P. (1996) [1968]. *The empty space: A book about the theatre. Deadly, holy, rough, immediate.* New York, NY: Simon & Schuster.

Cram, C. (2013). *On the floor.* Unpublished play.

Crenshaw, K. (2004). Intersectionality: The double bind of race and gender. *Perspectives Magazine.* Retrieved June 29, 2015, from http://www.american-bar.org/content/dam/aba/publishing/perspectives_magazine/women_per-spectives_Spring2004CrenshawPSP.authcheckdam.pdf

Cozolino, L. (2010). From neural networks to narratives: The quest for multilevel integration. In *The neuroscience of psychotherapy: Healing the social brain* (2nd ed., pp. 151–174). New York: Norton.

Ellis, C., Kiesinger, C., & Tillmann-Healy, L. (1997). Interactive Interviewing: Talking about emotional experience. In R. Hertz (Ed.), *Reflexivity and voice* (pp. 119–149). Thousand Oaks, CA: Sage.

Ellis, C., & Bochner, A. (2000). Autoethnography, personal narrative, reflexivity: Researcher as subject. In N. Denzin & Y. Lincoln (Eds.), *Handbook of qualitative research* (2nd ed., pp. 733–768). Thousand Oaks, CA: Sage Publications.

Ellis, C. (2007). Telling secrets, revealing lives: Relational ethics in research with intimate others. *Qualitative Inquiry, 13*(1), 3–29.

Emunah, R. (1994). *Acting for real.* New York: Brunner-Routledge.

Emunah, R. (2009). The integrative five phase model of drama therapy. In D. R. Johnson & R. Emunah (Eds.), *Current approaches in drama therapy* (2nd ed., pp. 37–64). Springfield, IL: Charles C. Thomas.

Emunah, R. (2015). Self-revelatory performance: A form of drama therapy and theatre. *Drama Therapy Review, 1*(1), 71–85.

Fox, J. (1999). Epilogue: The journey to deep stories. In H. Dauber & J. Fox (Eds.), *Gathering voices* (pp. 194–197). New Paltz, NY: Tusitala Publishing.

Gilligan, C. (1982). *In a different voice: Psychological theory and women's development.* Boston, MA: Harvard University.

Hodermarska, M. (2009). Perfume: A meditation on the countertransferential drama with babies who smell bad. *Arts in Psychotherapy, 36*(1), 39–46.

Hodermarska, M., Landy, R., Dintino, C., Mowers, D., & Sajnani, N. (2015). As performance: Ethical and aesthetic considerations for therapeutic theatre. *Drama Therapy Review, 1*(2), 173–186.

Jenkyns, M. (1996). *The play's the thing: Exploring text in drama and therapy.* New York: Routledge.

Johnson, D. (2009). Developmental transformations: Towards the body as presence. In D. R. Johnson & R. Emunah (Eds.), *Current approaches in drama therapy* (2nd ed., pp. 89–116). Springfield, IL: Charles C. Thomas.

Kilgannon, C. (2014). Therapist and patient share a theater of hurt. *The New York Times.* Available from http://www.nytimes.com/2014/11/06/nyregion/therapist-and-patient-share-a-theater-of-hurt.

LaFrance, M. (2013). The disappearing fourth wall: Law, ethics, and experiential theater. *The Vanderbilt Journal of Entertainment and Technical Law, 15*(3), 507–582.

Landy, R. J. (1993). *Persona and performance.* New York: Guilford.

Meldrum, B. (1999). The theatre process in dramatherapy. In A. Cattanach (Ed.), *Process in the arts therapies* (pp. 36–54). London: Jessica Kingsley.

Moreno, J. L., & Moreno, Z. T. (1969). *Psychodrama* (Vol. 1). Beacon, NY: Beacon House.

Pelias, R. J. (2008). Performative inquiry: Embodiment and its challenges. In J. G. Knowles & A. L. Cole (Eds.), *Handbook of the arts in qualitative research: Perspectives, methodologies, examples and issues* (pp. 185–194). Los Angeles: Sage Publications.

Ridout, N. (2009). *Theater & ethics.* New York: Palgrave Macmillan.

Rogoff, B. (2003). *The cultural nature of human development.* Oxford: New York.

Sajnani, N. (2012). The implicated witness: Towards a relational aesthetic in dramatherapy. *Dramatherapy, 34*(1), 6–21.

Sawyer, R. D., & Norris, J. (2013). *Duoethnography: Understanding qualitative research.* New York: Oxford University Press.

Scheff, T. (1979). *Catharsis in healing, ritual and drama.* Berkeley, CA: University of California.

Solnit, R. (2013). *The faraway nearby.* New York: Penguin.

Thompson, J. (2009a). Ah Pave! Nathiye: Respecting silence and the performances of not telling. In S. Jennings (Ed.), *Dramatherapy and social theatre: Necessary dialogues* (pp. 48–62). New York: Routledge.

Thompson, J. (2009b). *Performance affects: Applied theater and the end of effect.* New York: Palgrave Macmillan.

Thomson, P., & Jaque, S. V. (2011). Testimonial theatre-making: Establishing or dissociating the self. *Psychology of Aesthetics, Creativity, and the Arts, 5*(3), 229–236.

Yalom, V. (2004). Zerka Moreno on psychodrama. Retrieved from http://www.psychotherapy.net/interview/zerka-moreno

INDEX

© The Author(s) 2016
S. Pendzik et al. (eds.), *The Self in Performance*,
DOI 10.1057/978-1-137-53593-1